CW00646134

Ambush
on the Royal
Road

Surfacing memories
disrupt a therapist's career

Carolyn Shaw

To Edith,
with love from 'Carolyn'
June 2019

© Carolyn Shaw

This book is a work of non-fiction based on the experiences and recollections of the author. Names of people and places have been changed to protect the privacy of others.

Cover image:
American toad (*Bufo americanus*) hiding under a rock at the edge of a pond in central Virginia, ready to ambush passing prey. Cover design by Toby Matthews.

ISBN: 978-1-5272-3874-9

Printed and bound by
Holywell Press Ltd
Kings Meadow,
15-17 Ferry Hinksey Rd,
Oxford OX2 0DP

First published in 2019
by The Script Valet
scriptvalet@yahoo.com

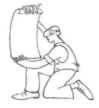

The interpretation of dreams is the royal road to a knowledge of the unconscious activities of the mind.

Sigmund Freud

For Christine

Acknowledgements

My heartfelt thanks are due to all the friends, relatives and professionals who supported me throughout the events related here – and also to those who have encouraged me to publish this account. Because of the nature of this book, they will remain anonymous.

A Note on the Title

The original title of this book was *Only My Truth*, for two reasons.

Firstly, no sooner had I begun to recover from the breakdown described here than my brother became ill with a brain tumour. He survived for eighteen agonising months. Six months after he died my husband was diagnosed with lung cancer. He, too, died – a little more than a year after my brother. The following year, one of my closest friends – now my husband – was driven to breakdown by events at work, and I was much taken up with supporting him through that.

Eventually he retired, and we married. It soon became clear that my own recovery process had been masked by all these events, and I wrote this story as a way of externalising it. Thus 'Only my Truth' also meant 'only *my* story', leaving out what had happened to my brother and to my first husband, as well as the events which preceded my second marriage.

The second reason for the original title was that almost all of the people concerned in the events of my childhood and adolescence had died before the memories began to surface: there was no-one apart from my brother – who had also been a child at the time – who could verify my story. In a more general sense, of course, this is true of all our memories: each one of us sees any story in which we have been involved from a different perspective.

Carolyn Shaw
December 2018

Contents

Dramatis Personae

(All names have been changed including the author's.)

Family

Carolyn

Hugh, Carolyn's father
Isabel, Hugh's mother
Cordelia, Hugh's sister

Deidre, Carolyn's mother
Nana, Deidre's mother and Carolyn's grandmother
William, Deidre's father
Jimmy, Deidre's brother
Paddy, Deidre's brother

Pete, Carolyn's brother
Jeanine, his partner

Hannah, Carolyn's Canadian partner

Jim, Carolyn's first husband
Kathy, Carolyn's daughter

Friends and colleagues

Jane and Franny, friends from University
Annie, a local friend
Harry Williams, theologian and monk
Toby, a colleague
Aileen, an old friend
Meg, one of Carolyn's clients

Figures from childhood

Dr O'Connor, the family GP
Miss Cowdry, RE teacher
Corinna Crisp, music teacher
Fred, the lodger
Perks, the verger

Doctors, Therapists, Clergy
from the time of the breakdown and recovery

Dr Gibson, a local GP
Mr O., psychotherapist
Patricia, Jungian analyst
Andrew, Jungian analyst and Carolyn's supervisor
Lydia and Gabriella, cranial osteopaths
Father Richard, parish priest

Foreword

We are born in relation,
we live in relation,
we die in relation.
There is, literally, no such human place
as simply 'inside myself'.
Nor is any person, creed, ideology,
or movement entirely 'outside myself'.

Carter Heyward

It's nearly thirty years ago now but I can still remember the two hour train journey across the Midlands for my first session with Carolyn. As for therapy, I was a virgin. As for life, I was far from innocent. Wrongly touched by others I was fragmented and worn down by oscillating cycles of reaching out and self-withdrawal. Whatever this therapy thing was, my whole life depended on it working. Now!

I spent the journey rehearsing my opening speech: 'This is me'; 'This is what you need to know'; 'Here's my check list'; 'When can we expect to see results?'

I knew precious little about Carolyn except that she came highly recommended. At least that's what they told me. In fact, that's *all* they told me. 'Boundaries' they said. Subversive as ever, I was on a mission to find out more.

I found the house, paced the street and on the stroke of five I rang the doorbell. On opening the door, she was smaller, more smiley and younger than I had imagined. The few steps from the door to her consulting room felt like entering Aladdin's Den: a cat occupying a place of honour; music open on a waiting piano; an icon of the Harrowing of

Hell on the mantelpiece. I took it all in and launched into my prepared script.

I needn't have bothered. The homely setting, the lived-in furniture, the sheer grace of being welcomed into a space which gave so much away about the stranger to whom I was invited to open up, told me I was Home! And that my battered and unscripted soul could come out of hiding.

It all happened thirty years ago and yet I remember that first therapeutic encounter so vividly and draw on it repeatedly in training others. 'You have heard so much about getting too close to people and maintaining your boundaries,' I tell my students, 'but how far are you willing to go to meet people where they are?' 'Boundaries have their place. Of course they do. But unless boundaries enable healing then the boundaries themselves may be unethical.'

My mantras continue: 'Don't confuse boundary *crossings* (intentional acts in the service of the client's wellbeing) with boundary *violations* (always and ever completely outlawed).

Sure, I trained as a therapist. But my real formation happened in that lived-in room where I was met, not by distant observation and analysis, but by a woman who (as this book relates) knew what it meant to be ambushed by returning memories and to face impending breakdown — and whose life so vitally depended on the Harrowing of Hell being a reality and not just a pretty image on the mantelpiece.

I knew on that very first meeting that my unbinding would take place in the company of a cloud of witnesses; my story would unfold within a community of poets and songwriters, story tellers and musicians, the crushed and the defeated, the half-risen and the thriving. This was hospitality in which deep could 'call to deep in the roaring of the waves' (Psalm 42.7).

In time the therapy ended but the healing continued. After some years I ventured back on that train to meet up with Carolyn but this time for tea and a chat as peers. It wasn't easy to come out of our previous roles but we persevered and went on to become life-long friends and to collaborate in teaching together.

Our friendship is one of the most exciting and durable boundary crossings I have ever made. Its lessons are many but they all boil down to one fundamental truth which is that therapist and client, helper and helped are fundamentally interdependent. In the words of the Aboriginal activists group, Queensland, in the 1970s,

If you have come to help me
You are wasting your time.
But if you have come
Because your liberation is bound up with mine
Then come, let us walk together.

If this book encourages even one professional helper to come out from behind his or her professional façade to question what often passes for professional wisdom then it will have been worth the raw, wounding pain that comes from hearing each other into speech.

Michael Paterson
Director, Institute of Pastoral Supervision
and Reflective Practice

PROLOGUE, 2011

'I WOULD LIKE YOU to try Prozac.'

Dr Gibson had been my doctor for twenty years and her suggestion was not unreasonable since I was weeping all over her office. I trusted her as a doctor, but drugs were another matter.

'I really don't like the idea,' I sniffed into my white cotton handkerchief.

'Why not?' she asked cheerfully, 'The whole town would come to a halt if it weren't for Prozac.'

'Well, OK, you can write out a prescription.' I told her, blowing my nose hard while she typed something into her computer.

'I can't guarantee to take it,' I added, cringing a little at my own self-importance.

Dr Gibson took a slip of green paper out of her printer, scrawled her signature and handed it to me.

'Take it.'

The pharmacy was across the road from the surgery, and as I handed over the prescription I started crying again. This was embarrassing, but it was also quite funny. They must be used to this, I said to myself. Then I went home and took the first one.

This is the story of a breakdown – or perhaps a break *through*, even a break *out*. What broke out of me was a story that had been locked away inside me for forty-four years. After my mother died, it simply found a way of being told.

It is a story I did not want to know. It made me feel

bad – so bad that as I write about it more than a decade later my body produces panic reactions and I am assaulted by voices: *What a self-obsessed old cow! Who wants to read about this disgusting stuff anyway? How could she be so unloving to her parents? Who does she think she is?*

These are voices that scream in the wake of people who seek to uncover memories of an attack. They are the last defences of a system desperate to protect itself from the truth. Even from this distance they can hurt, but as time goes on they shrivel into whimpering protest. They cannot bear your lack of desire to defend yourself against them, and impale themselves on the response, *So what? This is only my truth.*

When I took the first Prozac, however, I was not in search of any story, only desperate for some relief from the way I was feeling. For me, there was no knock at the door, no chance encounter. No-one asked, 'Do you remember ...?' I did not come on some arrangement of furniture, a smell, a striking clock or a twitch of a curtain that triggered a panic attack.

It was true that I had always been nervous at night, and liked to leave the bedroom door open so I could hear if anyone came up the stairs. But since leaving home – a vicarage – at seventeen, I had mastered sleeping through the night, travelling alone, keeping my weight steady. Now, at forty-eight, I had my own thriving therapy practice, a part-time lectureship in psychology, and some reputation as a writer. My daughter, Kathy, lived nearby with her boyfriend and she and her friends were in and out of the house most days. My husband, Jim, was absorbed in his graphic design business and the explosion in new software that almost daily opened up new possibilities. It was not a close marriage, but we both had full lives, and I loved mine. I had worked hard for it, and relished every day.

It had not always been easy to hold on to my work as a therapist during through the preceding two years while trying to support my mother through advanced alcoholism. Her death was followed by a winter of almost continuous flu alternating with exhaustion, but I weathered this too, getting up early to inhale Friar's Balsam before the first client arrived. It was understandable, I thought, that my resistance was low after my mother's protracted and crisis-ridden dying. But that was over now, and I had come through. So, in her own way, had she.

It was the following year, as the last Christmas of the millennium approached, that I had to admit to myself that I was not well.

As usual, I finished lecturing at the end of term, and continued seeing clients for another week. It was always a stressful time of year, working with twenty or so people through their feelings of dread about Christmas and/or the coming separation from me. As the last person left on Friday afternoon, I found that my own feelings of dread had taken over from my therapeutic self. I was used to feeling rough for a few days after stopping work and thought of it as a kind of bloodletting, allowing all that feeling to seep out of my system. Colleagues were often ill at these times: one had more than once been taken to hospital with all the symptoms of a heart attack. But this was different. Everything was suffused with a raw, despairing feeling. This was not just letting stress go. This was depression.

I knew a lot about depression: all my life I had watched my

mother drown in it and my brother Pete struggle with it. I lectured on it, wrote about it and worked with it – and I did not want to give it house room. The depression, however, did not seem interested in what I thought. Slowly, inescapably, it was shutting me down. All of a sudden my horizons were shrinking, and I had to force myself to go through the motions of preparing for Christmas, something I usually enjoyed. A high point of the week was when I made it into town – a twenty minute walk – to buy a present for my daughter Kathy. I recorded in my journal that I 'got it right' and this helped me feel 'a bit less despairing'. Christmas Day itself, I noted, was 'peaceful – quite good'.

There followed long empty days which I filled by preparing for a New Year party. From childhood I had felt that the turn of the year was best ignored: having survived the old year, why tempt fate by drawing attention to the arrival of the new one? That year, however, in a spirit of defiance, I threw a party for the new millennium. There was music, fireworks, great food. It was unlike me that I drank very little; my normal appetites were dampened down, and I was the one who was sober enough to give lifts to people who needed them when we had seen the New Year in. I drove home through the deserted streets and felt some kind of peace inside.

By morning that had vanished, and the first days of 2000 disappeared in a morass of bad feelings. I have always been sensitive to anniversaries and two years earlier I had spent this same first week of January – a window of opportunity before work began again – clearing my mother's house ready to sell it. Perhaps, I thought, I would feel this bad at this time every year for the rest of my life.

Then the long Christmas holiday was over, my clients returned, and term began. The life-saving routine was back in place.

I, less so. By February I was barely holding on.

People 'do' their depression in different ways, and mine was very physical. My face was steadily tightening up so that I could no longer smile, except as a kind of rictus. The tension around my forehead never let up. Nausea became a way of life, and sleeplessness simply non-negotiable. Every Thursday I wept throughout the half hour drive to the college where I taught, not knowing whether I could get through the day. Somehow I always managed to give my lectures and run my groups, but it took so much out of me that at the end of the day I sometimes had to stop in a layby on the way home so that I could give way to sobbing.

The more I shut down, the more insistent my dreams became. Something was demanding to be heard, and it felt as though my whole system – physical and mental – was fighting it off.

At half term, Jim and I went to Cornwall for a long weekend. I finished work early on the Friday, packed our things and sat in our large Victorian sitting room, staring at nothing while I waited for him to come back from the office. As usual, he was late, and what energy I had been able to muster for the journey steadily drained away.

After a while I became aware that Kathy and her boyfriend, Jack, had come in and were doing something at the far end of the room. Normally I would have been delighted to see them and offered tea or a drink, but I simply could not rouse myself to react to their presence –

even to look at them or say hallo. I became aware of Jack looking puzzled and asking Kathy, 'What's the matter?' and Kathy saying something about my not being well and not to worry. Even then I continued to stare into the fireplace, feeling vaguely shocked that she knew how ill I was. Soon they left, and Jim arrived. Somehow I managed to help him load the car, and we drove to Cornwall.

Our hotel stood at the top of a magnificent gorge running down to the sea. After dinner on the second night, enticed by a full moon, I followed a path that plunged down through a wood towards the sea. It followed a stream that ran among ferns and plants with huge, glossy green, timeless leaves. The whole thing was both enchanting and terrifying. Then everything suddenly opened out, and I was on the Cornish coast path where a few steps led down to a small bay with a sandy beach. The night was still and the sea barely rippled. So this was moonlight on water. As I stood and watched the eerie white light it made me think of my mother, as though it somehow explained her. The moonlight, I told myself, was dead and reflective, having no light of its own. Everything you saw came from another source.

That night I had a vivid dream, set around the church where my father had been vicar when I was a child:

> *I am an eight year old boy and I have arranged for detectives to arrest my father who has been sexually abusing me. We are all having tea, and I realise the arrest will be terrible for him and want to take him away – but it is too late. The matter is no longer in my hands. I go to the church and find the entrance is covered by curtains put there by the detectives and*

heave a sigh of relief: it will be safe to come here now. I unlock the door and let myself in. A woman's voice shouts 'Hallo, ducks!' and I realise there is a mad woman in one of the pews. I am terrified – and then I say to myself, 'It is only a mad woman'.

It was years since I had dreamed about my father, who had died back in 1985.

You could say that the dream in Cornwall was the 'initial dream' of the breakdown that was about to hijack my life.

As a therapist I was used to taking dreams seriously – my own and other people's – and this dream had a pattern that was familiar to me from working with people who had recovered memories of sexual abuse in childhood. In these dreams there is conflict between a persecutor, a victim and a rescuer, and there can be a lot interplay and ambiguity between these three. It may not be clear who is persecuting who, or whether the rescuer can be contacted or is capable of doing the job.

In my dream, I had organised detectives to remove my 'abusive' father, but I also did not want him to suffer. He had persecuted me, but I had set in motion a persecution of him, and it was too late to prevent him being taken away. I could no longer protect him from the 'detectives' – the healthy, protective aspects of myself. Although I had mobilised them, what they did was now beyond my control.

My father did not know it was me who had brought the detectives in. The scene at the tea table was dangerous for me because he might yet realise what I had done before they arrested him; and it was dangerous for him because they were going to take him away.

The detectives had also covered up the entrance to

the church — the church building of my childhood — and I was relieved: 'It is safe to come here now', I said to myself. With the entrance to the church covered so that I could not see inside, I could dare to go in. In other words, repression would protect me.

At the time of the dream, I had begun going to church again after a gap of nearly twenty years.

When, in the dream, I entered the church, I was recognised by a mad woman who at first scared me, until I realised 'It is only a mad woman' and there was no need to be afraid. Although I did not realise it I was on the brink of a madness which, although it was terrifying, was to prove necessary to my eventual survival. If the mad woman in the church represented my mad self, my reaction to her was correct.

In the dream I was a boy. This was not surprising since I spent much of my childhood pretending to be one. The boy in the dream was eight, an age when you can begin to take control of your life, and when issues of right and wrong and justice are particularly important. I still have very little memory of that part of my life.

When I had the dream, I did not know enough of my own story to analyse it as I have here, but I knew it was important and wrote it down in my journal. In five years of analysis with a Jungian therapist much had happened, but nothing like this dream about my father.

Nevertheless, I had suspected for some time that there was something about sexual abuse in my own story that I did not yet know. I had many characteristics that often go with a history of sexual abuse: I was an over achiever, scared of basements, prone to separation anxiety, and always concerned about weight problems.

Then there were the courses on sexuality I taught once a year with my colleague, Toby, for trainee clergy. Toby was a charismatic teacher, and always led the session on sexual abuse of children, drawing the group deeply into its implications. Usually someone in the group would start to cry during the discussion and tell us that, yes, everything Toby said was true. He or she had had an experience with a choir master, a priest, a teacher, a relative .....

I meanwhile would sit there in a state of rising panic, as though I, too, might be on the verge of such a revelation, though nothing ever actually surfaced. Yet I did not – and still do not – believe that my father sexually abused me, and though I had raked through what childhood memories I had, I found nothing.

Being unsure about this bothered me because in my job self-knowledge was all important. I knew I had been able to help people who recovered memories of abuse. I also knew that in five years of analysis I had not shirked exploration of my inner life, and had managed to reconcile many aspects of my past. My lifelong anger against my mother had retreated far enough for me to able to accompany her in her dying.

At the time of writing, I realise that I will never know the full story of what happened to me as a child. I can say, however, that I learned my own truth, and came to live with it.

Part 1
ORIGINS AND FIRST ENCOUNTERS

1

A Vicarage Childhood

VICAR HAS BABY DURING SERVICE. Thus the local paper announced my birth on a Sunday morning in May 1952.

This is how I liked to think of my arrival. Not a bed in a cramped bedroom with a woman in labour and other women in attendance, but my father standing up against the altar at the top of the chancel steps, his back to the people, a richly embroidered chasuble falling from his shoulders, his legs and feet hidden by folds of white: even as he raises his hands in prayer, I am born to him, appearing between his feet at the foot of the altar.

It was a powerful birth myth: not quite Athena emerging from the head of Zeus, but enough to keep my mother out of the picture.

The actual birth took place across the road from the church in a small suburban house. My grandmother, Nana, ran to announce my arrival with both thumbs in the air. 'Twins!' thought the congregation as they ambled out of church – or so my mother told me. But it was not so: just one little girl, a sister for my three year old brother, Pete.

As for the midwife, my mother, Deidre, said that she 'ran off' with the female doctor after I was born. This was my other birth myth: the two women cutting the umbilical cord, handing the baby over and kissing each other's lips before prancing hand in hand down the stairs and out of the front door.

As the second child, it always seemed to me that my arrival had been an intrusion on a world of conspiratorial delight shared between Pete and my mother. Even with him, however, feeding had been problematic. With Pete, my mother told me, she did not have enough milk. With me, she had abundant milk but it was 'too thin'. Who told her that? Was it I, already critical, who spat it out or failed to thrive? Was it those books that told mothers their babies must go for four hours and no more or less between feeds? Or was it her way of getting back to her own bottle without having to worry about what her babies were taking in?

Alcohol was already an important feature of Deidre's life. My father celebrated his first wedding anniversary in 1947 by writing a 'Staff Report' as 'General Lord Blogweed' on his wife (Lieutenant Was-Wiles) and mother-in-law (Col. Wiles) in which he noted of my mother, 'Particular praise is due for her ability to absorb alcohol and to sleep: the latter duties have been admirably carried out. ... Character: A little lovey gorm'. Of her mother, who lived with them, he says, 'Brave in the face of Frost, Electric Cuts and Labour Government .... Character: Quite a bird.'

My father was never in the army, being exempt from call-up as a trainee priest. His own father had also been exempt in World War One as a Civil Servant. Of my mother's brothers, one was disabled, and the other a policeman, so our family was curiously untouched by war – another thing that set our experience apart from those around us. There had been devastation and loss on my mother's side, but for different reasons.

The eccentric document of 'General Lord Blogweed' expresses something of the oddity of my parents' marriage – though it was a long and successful one. As my brother Pete put it, there were two sides to the family – posh (my father's) and poor (my mother's). When my parents declared their engagement it must have been a shock on both sides.

The 1901 census shows both my grandmothers at the age of around fifteen. My father's mother, Isabel, is on holiday in a hotel in Bournemouth with her parents and two sisters (one of whom became a nun and the other a missionary); my mother's mother, Beatrice, was already a 'general domestic' in service in Barnes. One thing they had in common is that they both married relatively late for the time – Isabel at thirty to a man four years younger, and Beatrice at twenty-nine to a man twenty-five years older (though he had lied to her about his age and she thought the age gap was fifteen years, only discovering the truth after his death).

The only one of her siblings to marry, Isabel had great personal wealth. Unable to compete with her sisters in piety, she could – and did – nevertheless produce a son, Hugh, for the priesthood. He was sent to boarding school from the age of seven.

Beatrice had three children, my mother being the youngest. The oldest, James, was blind and epileptic following a botched forceps delivery. He was eleven and my mother seven when Beatrice's husband, an alcoholic, died on the streets leaving behind a string of failed businesses. This was long before we had the NHS or a welfare state. She worked all hours in whatever jobs she could get – domestic service, factory work and so on. There were constant house moves, each one involving for my mother the immortalised loss of some treasured object. It was she who inherited her father's poetic imagination and addictive tendency, and she idealised him, the family story becoming for her a potent cocktail of guilt and regret.

Neither of my parents, then, could be said to have had much of a childhood. Without the church it is unlikely that they would ever have met. Hugh's first curacy in 1943 was in the parish where Deidre was a keen church attender and ran the Brownies. Their intimacy deepened in the air raid shelters, where she was taken with the way he sat and knitted dishcloths for the war effort. They fell in love and married, and because my mother could not bear to leave her mother, Beatrice came too. While the past was ever present for Deidre, Beatrice rarely spoke of it – or her husband – to her grandchildren.

I have no doubt that both my parents longed for Pete and me to be happy and secure in our childhood, and we certainly led much more comfortable lives than they ever did. But the intergenerational demons were not so easily tamed.

I was one year old when my father became vicar of a parish in a prosperous London suburb. Let's call it St George's. My parents, Beatrice – now Nana – and Pete and I moved to a seven bedroom Victorian vicarage, and there we stayed until shortly after my twelfth birthday.

Having started life as a general domestic, Nana willingly took on the care of the vicarage, making the kitchen, larder and scullery her domain. She cooked and scrubbed and knitted and darned, and threaded the knicker elastic. On Tuesdays she took Pete and me across the road to collect her pension, from which she gave each of us sixpence to buy sweets. Otherwise she rarely went out, apart from the weekly family visit to my uncle's residential hospital. My father always referred to her as 'Cousin'.

Hugh was a high church Anglican priest of his time: public school, Oxford, Cuddesdon. Five foot nine inches tall, he weighed seventeen stone and had a tonsure of black curly hair. He was never far away from a cigarette, and wherever he was or had been there was the comforting scent of tobacco. His mornings were spent in his study behind a kneehole desk on which stood a telephone, an inkstand, various papers and a cut glass ashtray the size of a tea plate. Two armchairs faced each other across the fireplace and in the corner stood a square dining table covered with a grey tapestry cloth. Here stood a magnificent steel grey typewriter on which, by special arrangement, I was allowed to type the newspaper I regularly produced for my toys. Otherwise, the study was sacrosanct and entered by invitation only – and even then after knocking.

After lunch, my father took his nap in the sitting room, stretched out in an armchair and snoring loudly, before setting forth on his pastoral visits. He disliked conflict and cut an amiable and reassuring figure in the parish. From time to time he would announce that he was going to 'church' a woman. Whatever this was, I did not like the sound of it.

Deidre did not go out to work, except for short bursts of supply teaching (she had trained as a teacher before marriage). Since Nana did the bulk of the housework and

14

there was also a weekly cleaner she was relatively free to write and paint, as she wanted to do – but seemed always under pressure to find time for these things. She liked being a vicar's wife, but from the early days of their marriage she was prone to stay up late at night and was always tired in a way that would now be recognised as depression but which we then took for granted – as in 'General Lord Blogweed's' report. One curious memory of her is that her handbag was always enormously heavy. If anyone picked it up to pass it to her they would exclaim, 'What on earth have you got in here? Rocks?' She would reply that it contained my father's love letters from before they were married. It is a matter of regret that I never saw these letters, but however ardent they may have been it is hard to believe they were that heavy. Perhaps they were a front for a hip flask.

Apart from Nana who did not believe in God, our lives revolved around church. Parishioners came and went from my father's study and some – much to my disgust – hung around the kitchen. We ate fish on Fridays, gave up chocolate for Lent, went carol singing at Christmas, held the summer fete in our garden and said prayers each night before going to bed. Every Sunday was a little Easter, every sleep a little death. Pete and I learned the Sunday Collects each week like Victorian children – or at least I did. I have a vague memory of Pete just stopping, and of my father's silent but angry reaction.

At seven, first Pete and then I were invited into the study to be taught Latin. This was an echo of Hugh's own upbringing. It was at seven that he had been sent away to prep school and had there begun Latin himself, just like

Winston Churchill, whom he so closely resembled. We were never allowed to forget that we had been spared boarding school with its cold showers and its beatings (Hugh had the honour of having received more than a hundred strokes), the toilets without doors and the terrible food. The Latin lessons were no more a success with Pete than the weekly Collects had been, but when my turn came I perched on the armchair across from my father, chirpily reciting *Amo, amas, amat; mensa, mensa, mensam*. Unlike Churchill, I found no absurdity in it, only a reassuring sense of order.

To this day, however, my childhood memories are few. Although I went to St George's every Sunday and feast day for the first twelve years of my life, I can hardly remember being there. There are vignettes, no more: throwing a tantrum when I had to wear a skirt instead of shorts; standing beside my mother in the front pew as she swayed off into sleep and seeing her jerk awake just before she dropped the hymn book; the little bell tinkling way up the steps in the sanctuary while my father grasped the edge of the altar and genuflected three times; Pete as 'boat boy' in cassock and cotta, holding the silver boat-shaped container of incense, processing in and out with the servers, the heavy hand of one of the men on his shoulder; the longing to be allowed to do likewise. At ten I was given a satiny and voluminous white dress – I was already the normal weight of an adult – in which I was confirmed and received my first communion. The dress is what I remember.

Thereafter I joined my mother and Pete on occasional excursions to a city centre church where there were wooden cubicles for confession. I prepared for these outings carefully, kneeling by my bed and consulting the various possibilities for sin offered in the leather bound

Manual of Catholic Devotion given to me by my aunt Cordelia as a confirmation present. Had I taken God's name in vain? Had I been disrespectful in church? Had I wilfully doubted any teachings of the Church? Wished evil on anyone? Indulged in boasting or vainglory? Gradually, I compiled my personal 'sin list'.

On arrival at All Saints, we sat waiting with other penitents. Eventually my mother would usher me towards a vacant box. I entered and knelt beside a grille behind which a priest was dimly visible. He said the opening prayers, I confessed my sins, and received a penance – so many 'Our Fathers' or 'Hail Mary's – and absolution. The relief of being absolved was intoxicating. On our return home, my mother ceremoniously lifted the lid of the kitchen stove and we all dropped our lists in, watching it flare up in response.

St George's was the high point of Hugh's career. When the time came to move on, it being considered bad form for a vicar to stay beyond ten years, there was a flurry of excitement about possible futures. My father emerged as a man without ambition who loved pastoral work: a good parish priest but not bishop material. This was a great disappointment to my mother, who affirmed Hugh's lack of ambition as a sign of holiness while lamenting it as a waste of talent.

Around this time she had a story published in a women's weekly magazine: a dowdy woman joins a parish and is ostracised while they prepare with great excitement for a visit from the bishop. On the great day the dowdy woman turns out to be the bishop's sister: he greets her with great affection while the parishioners are overcome with chagrin. Deidre was fond of secrets with happy endings of this kind.

Not only did my father not become a bishop, but his next parish was much further out of London. For my parents it turned out to be a good move. For Pete and me it was more of a challenge. Since we both had scholarships to private day schools in the city centre, our daily journey time was increased by about an hour each way. Neither of us mixed much with the parishioners of the new church, Holy Trinity, though Pete continued to be a server. We were not popular, being the vicar's children as well as going to posh schools. Pete made a better job of it than I did. He had two advantages: not being fat as I was (twelve stone at the age of twelve, fifteen stone at fifteen), and having copied Deidre's working class accent rather than Hugh's Oxford one which I had adopted. I briefly joined the Guides but left after being threatened with a mallet.

Though I do not remember it I must, however, have joined the choir, because a year or two after we arrived, I was due to go on a choir outing with Mr Pimm, the organist. It was Saturday morning and the thought of getting on a coach with all those people filled me with dread. As usually happened on such occasions I developed diarrhoea, and announced that I could not go.

'OK,' said my mother, 'but you need to tell Mr Pimm yourself.' My insides already beginning to settle, I marched to my father's study and looked up the number.

'Hallo' said a girl's voice.

'Is Mr Pimm there please?'

'No. It's his daughter. Who is speaking please?'

'This is Carolyn Nash.'

'Yes?'

'I was ringing to say I am not feeling very well and

can't come on the choir outing. Please could you tell Mr Pimm?'

'Mr Pimm won't be going anywhere, He has just had a massive heart attack'

Click.

It was typical that my dubious malaise should be so upstaged, leaving me feeling guilty and mean. It was also how, at fourteen, I became my father's organist.

All my life I had longed to work for my father, begging to be allowed to file his papers, type his letters, bring order to his world. I had dreams of being a Parish Worker, cycling around the homes of the sick and the poor with a little badge on my chaste blue jacket. It was then unheard of for girls to serve in the sanctuary. So insistent was I in wanting to join Pete amongst the servers that when I was six my parents let me dress up in a cassock and cotta for a photograph which was then displayed on the mantelpiece. I hated that photograph – a symbol to me of everything I was not allowed to be. Now the organ loft became my province.

It took some time to realise that even so, my father would never really tell me what he thought or felt about anything. It was as though at some stage in his life he had drawn a line across himself at around chest height and vowed never to go below it. Once, in a rare burst of communication, he admitted as much. All his life, he had wanted to be a priest. Only once, he told me, did he question that sense of vocation. While a student at Oxford he one day stood by the window of his room, looked out over the High, and asked himself whether he might not do something completely different. The answer came back, no, and he never questioned it again. Like the adolescent Jung, I raged inwardly against my father's refusal to entertain any form of doubt, and pressed him with questions, but it was always turned into some kind of kind of joke, or a simple refusal to discuss whatever it was.

There were many weddings, for example, where I played the organ and he officiated. They disturbed me as I could not imagine being willing to make such extravagant promises to anyone. One day, on the way home I asked him, 'You always preach the same sermon at weddings. Is that what you really believe about marriage?'

'Well, you always play the same music,' he countered, and that was that.

These attempts at dialogue reached a head when I was fifteen, and choosing my A level subjects. I wanted to do what was then called 'Scripture' A level, alongside Latin, Greek and Music. I even had visions of myself as a theologian, poring over ancient texts in dark Oxford libraries. Miss Cowdry, the Scripture teacher, was lean and intense, with long dark hair and large tortoiseshell glasses. She rode a motorbike in leathers, and was quite unlike any of the women at church – or indeed the other women who taught at my rather exclusive girls' school. At the end of the summer term she gave me an exciting looking reading list full of names I had never heard of: Bultmann, Bonhoeffer, Tillich ....

I made the mistake of showing it to my father.

Without a word to me he went straight to the school. 'I am not having my daughter taught heresy,' he growled at Miss Cowdry. Then he came home and told me that I would not be doing Scripture at A level.

Miss Cowdry tried to persuade me to defy him, but I could not find it in myself to do that. I settled for the other three.

In particular, I was determined to take Music not just because I loved it but because it was taught by my organ teacher, Miss Crisp, a mysterious and charismatic woman in her mid-thirties. She was tall and slim, with narrow hips and honey coloured hair which she kept short and straight. Her eyes were grey, and she wore eye shadow to match whatever she was wearing, along with pale lipstick and dark foundation. Her voice was deep and a little husky, her accent polished and her speech clipped. She stuttered on 'c's and had a nervous twitch of her bushy eyebrows. Every morning she arrived at the school in a white convertible MG.

Never had organ playing been so popular as it became during Miss Crisp's time – or so well taught. Currents of desire fizzed around her. Even my mother fell for the way she moved her hands when she was conducting at a school concert.

I persuaded my parents to ask her at the parents' evening if I could do Music A level. My mother reported that she paused, stared into space for a few moments, and then replied, 'Yes, I think she could do it.'

For all my chosen subjects, the classes were tiny – three of us for Greek, five for Music and about ten for Latin. It was bliss, and I worked extremely hard. My dreams of being an Oxford theologian gave way to dreams of becoming a Cambridge musicologist, Miss Crisp having been at Newnham. My adult life would be spent sitting in an ivory tower unearthing old manuscripts, and then editing them so that they could come alive for the first time in centuries.

Despite the relish with which I approached my work, I was also extremely anxious. There was a constant throbbing pain under my ribs, and I had frequent mouth ulcers and fits of vomiting. When I finally produced a black stool, my mother said darkly that this was 'not a good sign' and took me to the doctor.

Visits to the doctor were something I avoided if possible, not because of the doctor but because as the vicar's family we were allowed to jump the queue of obviously sick people waiting miserably to see him. Just before we left home my mother would ring the surgery and announce we were coming: we would then walk straight in to his office under the resentful eyes of everyone in the waiting room. Doctor O'Connor was an affable Irishman who spoke very fast and very softly, with a mournful expression that implied death was imminent. He referred me to the hospital, where I was given a barium meal and examined by a consultant. At least this man spoke loud and clear, diagnosing a duodenal ulcer and a congested liver.

'I don't know what to say to you,' he remarked, looking at my results, 'You have the digestion of a fifty year old business man, but since you are a fifteen year old schoolgirl, I do not know what to say.'

He prescribed antacids and suggested eating little and often – and perhaps altogether less. Until then I had been in the habit of eating neither breakfast nor lunch, but one large meal on arriving home from school, and another at bed time. Now I began taking my own diet in hand: the ulcer cleared up completely, though I continued to struggle with keeping my weight under control.

At home, Nana had become increasingly frail and was no longer able to look after the house – a sprawling vicarage. Without her, nothing kept back the tide of miscellaneous objects, dirty dishes and generalised mess that seemed to crawl out of the walls. At one end of the kitchen an enormous dresser was almost invisible behind old newspapers and magazines, books, crockery, cooking utensils, pens, broken toys, ornaments – and a complete set of plastic models in different sizes of Fred the Flour-Grader from Home Pride flour – perhaps the only complete set of anything in the entire house.

My mother, meanwhile, had made a life-changing discovery. The GP, Dr O'Connor, became concerned that my father was still seventeen stone and approaching fifty, and prescribed some of the new miracle slimming pills. Hugh took them for a week, lost no weight and gave up, but Deidre, always worried about her weight though she was not fat, gave them a try. The little yellow pills gave her an exquisite rush of energy, and from then on she was never without some in her handbag. She also gave them to Pete and me when we were revising for exams so that we could stay awake at night. I only tried them a couple of times because I had trouble sleeping anyway, but they were certainly effective. Every few weeks she would ring up for a fresh prescription for my father, who never took them and whose weight never varied.

Always a night drinker, she also began to drink more openly – with the curate, the lodger, Pete and his friends – anyone, in fact who was happy to sit around the kitchen table and consume whisky. I would have none of it, and sat upstairs in my bedroom learning Greek verbs and chewing Ryvita.

Nana's room, also upstairs, was a refuge. It was warm and dimly lit, and I liked to sit on her bed and chat or watch telly, or simply hold her hand. She was still able to sit up in bed and knit, and at Christmas she gave me a little drawstring bag she had knitted from bright blue wool. In it were five shillings from 1952, my birth year. Pete had a similar bag, with five shillings from 1949. She had no money beyond her pension, and these little bags were farewell presents: her particular legacy to us.

By New Year 1969, she had pleurisy and pneumonia, and my mother warned me to listen out for the 'death rattle' in her breathing, or signs of approaching death like plucking at the sheets. She and I took it in turns to sleep on the sofa in Nana's room in case she died in the night. On 8 February, a Saturday, I woke up on the sofa to see Deidre leaning over the bed and crying, and trying to push Nana's teeth back in place so that she would not settle into *rigor mortis* with her mouth sunk in. It had been one of my nights 'on' and she had died, and I had slept through it. Hugh was away at early Mass, so I went down to meet him at the front door and told him what had happened. He made a kind of grunt, but I could not ignore the relief on his face. The district nurse, a parishioner, came to lay her out. I offered to help, and was struck by her refusal of the offer on the grounds it wasn't really appropriate. I felt embarrassed and confused, but also somehow cared for.

The next day Pete and I were delegated to empty the grate in the sitting room so there should be no warm coals before the undertakers brought in Nana's body in an open coffin. People came and said goodbye, and wept a bit. I remained stony and tearless until the morning of the funeral, when I sobbed upstairs while the undertakers banged the nails into the coffin lid. Nevertheless, I played the organ for the funeral, as I had done for my other grandparents, my father taking the service.

Nana was buried in our churchyard, and for months afterwards I had dreams in which she turned up in the kitchen not knowing she was dead and had to be taken back to her grave. I desperately wanted to dig her up so that I could hold her hand again. In Music A Level class we were doing Berlioz's *Symphonie Fantastique*, which we listened to on a record. The tolling bell in 'The March to the Scaffold' seared my brain. It was some comfort to notice Miss Crisp notice that I was upset.

That summer I sat my A levels and came out with straight A's.

2

The Choice

At school, the demand for organ practice times had grown, thanks to the attraction of Miss Crisp, so she now gave me lessons at St Andrew's, a city church where she was organist. She drove me there in her white MG after school on Wednesdays. At home in the parish there was competition for my post, a local boy who was a keen and proficient organist, and it was clear that my father wanted to encourage him by giving him my job. Feeling hurt and ousted, I soon began to act as Miss Crisp's assistant at St Andrew's on Sundays. The journey from home took the best part of two hours.

St Andrew's was a completely different experience of church from my father's parish. There was a professional paid choir and a vicar who was given to long and stirring sermons about the value of war in fostering community spirit, and whose car displayed a sticker: 'Think Navy, think deep.' It was also was my first encounter with Matins, which was not without repercussions at home. One day I was asked about St Andrew's by my aunt Cordelia, who felt responsible for my soul. When she realised that I was spending Sunday mornings at Matins instead of Mass she was appalled: I was allowing myself to 'fall out of communion'. It worried me that she was so concerned, and I started going once a week to the early Mass said daily by my father. I liked this because there was none of the fuss that surrounded the Sunday service – just the Mass itself. One evening at supper, as I nibbled a Ryvita and enviously watched the rest of them tuck in to eggs and bacon and beer, I made the mistake of saying so. My father's face lit up and he turned to my mother and said, 'The child is an incipient saint.' From then on I went less, and eventually stopped going altogether.

St Andrew's was near Soho, and seeing prostitutes on the street I bought myself a book, *The Oldest Profession*, to try to learn more about them. My father asked me what I was reading, and then why on earth I should want to read such a book.

'I see these people on the streets in London, and I want to understand more about them.'

'That's not what you should be doing.'

'What should I be doing?'

'You should pray and pass on.'

Although A levels were over, there was one more term at school when I was to study with Miss Crisp for Oxbridge entrance in Music. In August, I stayed with her for three nights so I could attend a course at the Royal College of Organists while my family started the three week summer holiday in Devon. She lived in a high ceilinged flat with a large room overlooking the garden. It was extremely clean and tidy, and with its muted colours, soft lighting and sparse furnishings seemed to me the apotheosis of style. There was no piano, but there was a small spinet – and there were no knick-knacks anywhere, even in the kitchen. I was still very upset about Nana dying, and on the last afternoon, just before I went to join my family in Devon, we sat in the living room and I talked about how I used to sit with Nana and hold her hand, and how much I longed to hold her hand again.

I was in the armchair, and Miss Crisp was lounging on the divan by the window, not saying much. Suddenly she spoke: 'Come over here.'

I looked over at her, surprised.

'Come over here. Come on.'

I went and sat on the divan and she took my hand and held it. We sat there for a while like that, and then it was time to go and catch my train.

In Devon I spent the days wandering on the beach. I realised I was being seduced, that I desperately wanted to be seduced, that I did not really know what this meant, and that I would burn for ever in hell if I allowed myself to be seduced by a woman. I peered endlessly into rock pools while I thought about it. By the end of the holiday there was only one possible conclusion: Miss Crisp *was* worth burning in hell for.

Back in London I spent a delicious autumn term studying for Oxbridge, eventually gaining a minor organ scholarship at Oxford. Then, the day after I left school, in December, Miss Crisp invited me to meet her for a walk. She picked me up in her car outside Edgware Road tube station.

The MG had been replaced by a maroon Renault 4, with bench seats in the front and a gear stick that came out from the dashboard. It was cold and she was wearing black bobbly woollen gloves. She clasped my hand briefly when I got in, and then drove to Regent's Park. As we arrived it started to rain very heavily, so she parked and we sat in the car, the rain coming down in sheets around us. To my astonishment Miss Crisp started to cry. I reached over and put my hand on the back of her neck.

'What's the matter?' I asked.

'I don't want your life to be like mine'

This was a mysterious comment. All I longed for in the world was to be like her – free, self-supporting, a 'wealthy working woman' as she used to say. After a while she reached inside my jeans and I had a moment of recognition: *Oh, it's that.*

Afterwards we drove through the rain to her flat and spent the night there – and the next – and I learned to call her Corinna. When I finally walked back into the vicarage, it was as though my father did not recognise me. He walked past me in the hall, then turned round and looked at me.

'You are beautiful', he remarked in great surprise.

That Christmas holiday Corinna and I redecorated her flat and made love incessantly surrounded by the smell of paint and oranges. I wandered back and forth between Hampstead and the vicarage, and dumped all my friends. I was blissfully happy.

'If only we could get married,' I said one day

'We'll go mad if we think about that,' replied Corinna.

She pointed out that it was only a couple of years since, if we were men, we could have gone to prison for what we were doing. She relayed this with such intensity that it did not occur to me that since I was only seventeen, she would have been the one to go to prison if we were men. The very thought made me feel somehow noble and extraordinary. And I spoke to no one, no one at all.

Corinna was like Laurence Durrell's Justine: 'Her gift was misapplied in being directed towards love .... But those she harmed most she made fruitful. She expelled people from their old selves.' This Corinna certainly did for me. She taught me how to wash up (glasses first, then cutlery, plates, saucepans); how to make a cheese sauce (always take the *roux* off the heat before adding the milk) and liquidise soup; to use Tampax; to change gear in her Renault 4. All my life I had lived on the edge of London, but she showed me the centre – the art galleries, theatres, concert halls. We frequented a little Italian coffee shop in Tottenham Court Road to drink frothy coffee in shallow Pyrex cups, and held hands under the table: Corinna always ate her froth with a spoon. With her, I read Iris Murdoch, listened to the Beatles and Dusty Springfield, played chess. It was Corinna who introduced me to the countryside, bird watching, and long walks in the country.

Alas for me, I had not bargained to start burning in hell so soon. It was only a few weeks before Corinna began playing me off against lovers of both sexes. One Sunday night we were driving back to her flat after an Evensong where we had performed a particularly complex anthem, I playing the organ and she conducting the choir.

'I was thinking during choir practice,' she remarked later as we headed down Tottenham Court Road, '"there is no-one in this room I haven't slept with".'

It had not occurred to me that Corinna slept with men as well as women and I ran through the choir members in my mind. Yes, I could imagine Marc, or Paul, or Felicity. But surely not Alice? Surely not Ian? But this was all in the past and did not really concern me. Then it turned out that there was a male lover right now and she was thinking of marrying him. At first incredulous, I quickly accepted my position as second best since sometimes I was still allowed to sleep with her. When the lover was around I silently suffered jealous torments at my parents' house. Still I spoke to nobody.

One evening I came in late when my father was washing up the supper things in his shirt sleeves, as he always did before he went to bed. I decided to confide in him, and sat down at the kitchen table.

'I've been having a terrible time,' I said.

My father picked up his cigarette from the ashtray on the draining board and took a deep drag. 'Yes,' he replied, 'the tube can be bad at this time of night.'

I went to bed.

In October I went up to Oxford. From then on Corinna refused to sleep with me anymore. 'You've bulldozed me into this relationship,' she accused me, 'and now you won't let me out of it.'

The male lover had emigrated but she now said she had a regular female lover and could not sleep with both of us. The identity of the lover was none of my business. It was, she told me, time I found someone my own age, preferably male. Again the choice was to accept this or lose her altogether, so I accepted it: she remained the centre of my life and I went back in the Christmas and Easter vacations to play the organ at St Andrew's. There was never any sign of the new lover, and in my first summer vacation we walked the Pennine Way together: two hundred and fifty miles in three weeks. She spent months planning it out, arranging accommodation in youth hostels and bed and breakfasts. My mother, with her usual knack of naming what could never be discussed, expressed horror that we were going to stay in B&Bs: 'You might end up sharing a room with a raving lesbian or something,' she said. *If only ...*

I loved the walking, the constant moving on, and there was a kind of simplicity in the fact that we no longer slept together, though we often shared a room. We walked all day, often in pouring rain, and in the evenings we read or played chess. It was in the third week, as we were making our way along Hadrian's Wall, that a name came into my head: the name of Susanna Taylor. Susanna Taylor was several years below me at school, and in fact she was still there. She had stood out from the other girls right from the beginning, and she was very musical. By now she would be around sixteen or seventeen...

As usual we were greeted at a farmhouse with a large and delicious supper. I waited until we were settled in our twin beds and had put the lights out.

'It's Susanna, isn't it', I said into the darkness. There was a short silence.

'How did you know?'

'I just knew. How could you?' Another silence. Then,

'She is so insistent. I don't know how to get out of it.'

Susanna, she went on to say, had been raped as a child by her uncle. Then no more was said by either of us.

This was a first-hand encounter with what Freud calls reaction formation. A feeling is so strong that you dare not let yourself feel it because of the damage you might do to someone you love. It therefore gets suppressed into the unconscious and what you experience is its opposite. All through breakfast the next morning I watched myself being as nice as anyone could be to Corinna: passing the toast, even letting her have the last precious piece (we got very hungry walking). I walked very hard and fast that day and during the days that followed.

Eventually we reached the Plough in Kirk Yetholm and claimed our free half pint for anyone who finished the Pennine Way.

Still I said nothing to anyone and continued to see Corinna whenever I could. A few weeks into the following autumn term, however, the mother of yet another girl at the school who was obsessed with Corinna discovered her relationship with Susanna and saw an opportunity to be rid of her. The headmistress called Corinna in and invited her to resign. By Christmas she had abandoned us all and gone to live abroad. I could not imagine how I would live without her.

Nevertheless, I did survive. At least I now felt able to confide in two fellow students about my lost love. They were both kind, and have remained friends for life. I was not ready to accommodate what one of them said – 'She sounds like rather an unpleasant person' – but the comment stayed with me and as time went on I would sometimes try it out to see if it made sense yet.

The rest of my time at Oxford was spent in a daze. Although I had entered on Music I had switched to Philosophy and Psychology, neither of which, it turned out, made sense to me in the form they were taught at Oxford. Hours were spent in the Radcliffe Science library trying to understand articles – for which I had neither appetite nor background – on the neuro-physiology of cats, rats and other animals, octopuses included. One moment in the second year sticks in my mind. I was sitting among the library stacks at a dark wooden table. A glimmer of late afternoon sun was falling on its polished surface. The paper in front of me was by Konrad Lorenz, on imprinting in chicks.

Scanning the article in my usual state of half-comprehending boredom I suddenly found my attention caught. I read that when a chick hatches from the egg, it 'imprints' on the first moving object it sees. Normally this object is its mother, but if the moving object is something else – even a human being – the bird irreversibly has a lifelong image of itself as that object stamped on its brain. In human terms it sees in the imprinted object its own nature, what it is destined to become. This takes place across many different species of bird. It was Lorenz who established that human-imprinted birds will not enter into courtship rituals in the wild because they are confused about their own identity.

This information hit me like a kick in the stomach. Here was what had happened to me with Corinna. At fourteen I had sat in the school hall and heard her give an organ recital. The moment she stepped out from behind the organ screen to accept the applause, at a distance of thirty feet away and never having exchanged a word, I knew this person was necessary to me – the 'imprinting' happened and was apparently irreversible. This insight did not help – if anything it made it more painful – but at that time it was the only sense in which I could begin to understand I had been duped.

At Oxford I had little sense of connection to anything or anyone, except my two close friends who kept me alive, and it was as though I had no past. I could remember more or less nothing about church, my upbringing, or almost anyone I had ever known. Short of money, I one day emptied Nana's five shillings into my purse and threw away the bag, telling myself contemptuously, *They are only money.* As for churches, apart from my duties in the college chapel I kept well away: the sound of organ or choral music hurt too much in any case. In the curious way that human beings have I continued to see, interact with and worry about my parents and Pete and my aunt Cordelia: I just had no sense of belonging with them.

Somehow I came out with a respectable degree. There were also a few short lived and disastrous attempts to go out with men, all of whom I treated badly, but I did manage, as I put it to myself, to get rid of my virginity. This, after all, seemed to be what Corinna had expected of me.

During the final spring term it occurred to me that I would have to support myself after the end of that summer, and I applied for a job as a social work assistant in a London hospital. By autumn I had my own spacious office and phone extension, along with a white coat for visiting the wards. The job was alternately very exciting and unbearably depressing. I loved the atmosphere of the hospital and apart from expecting an IRA bomb to go off every time I went into the Tube, also loved being in central London.

Being unqualified, I was given the old people, the amputees and the drunks. The real social workers dealt with miscarriages, cancer and everything in between. I found myself strangely at home with the drunks, became very attached to the old people – many of whom were referred to us as 'disposal' problems because they were not well enough to go home – and forced myself to visit the amputees, on the basis that it must be worse for them than it was for me. Though I did not know it, I was being introduced to listening skills, casework and managing boundaries. Boundaries were not my strong point. The head of department was not happy, one evening when she swept through Casualty, to see me sitting with a drunk holding his hand. But I was dynamic, and at Christmas I gained glory for the department by stepping in and conducting the hospital's carol service (rather well) when the conductor fell ill at the last minute. I was sorry when the job – a training post only for a year – came to an end.

Then I, too, fled the country, and spent four years on the west coast of Canada, teaching music in private schools. Here I met Hannah. She was not Corinna, but she was a beautiful woman only a few years older than me who taught me a great deal about love and being a woman. Shortly after we moved in together I had a dream:

> *I am on my way back to the flat I share with Hannah on Vancouver Island, when I am suddenly confronted by St George's church. I start screaming, 'No! No! It is not here! It's in England! My parents were never on Vancouver Island!' People around reassure me. 'No, it's just a clever replica – a tourist attraction. St George's really is in England.' I am in a state of panic and shaking all over.*
>
> *Hannah's father – a painter – comes to me and says, 'You must paint this out. It's the only way you'll ever get over it. He fetches me his best drawing board and easel.*
>
> *As I sit down to paint the sun is setting, and the scene becomes a flat oceanic sea ….*

3

Benefits of Amnesia

AMNESIA is a strange and powerful thing.

In Canada I achieved the life I had wanted ever since I met Corinna: a good job, money, a lover, a modern flat that we kept tidy and clean. Hannah was slim and blonde and very feminine, and it was her first time with a woman. I loved her body, her moods, her softness, and the way she knew about things I did not: hair dye, ear piercing, underwear, how to make a home nice and orderly the way ours was. Our life together was everything I had come six thousand miles to find. I loved visiting her parents who lived in a spacious house on a small holding further up the island. Her father let me mow the lawn and help him with the income tax like any son-in-law. Her mother bustled and chatted and produced home-made cakes and five-thirty high tea. At night when I could not sleep, Hannah would hold me in her arms and tell me stories of her childhood, of family picnics, visits to aunties, campsites where bears rooted in the garbage, shopping with her older sisters. Slowly, steadily, these stories seeped in amongst my night terrors and began to push them aside.

All the same, a strange thing started happening to me. The first time I noticed it, we were on our way to visit

Hannah's parents. Hannah was at the wheel of her little blue hatchback. I liked watching her drive. She had decided to take the scenic route past Tzuhalem, a sacred mountain enclosed in a reservation. I was angry about the Canadians' attitude to the indigenous population: having taken their land and destroyed their way of life, they now complained the original inhabitants were idle and drunk. Hannah wanted me to see that the government at least supplied protected spaces for them.

We rounded a bend, and Hannah pointed out to me the low rounded hill which was the sacred mountain. Like so much of Vancouver Island it had an air of brooding silence. It was only when we were close that we could see the wire fence and the people who lived behind it. A few hundred yards beyond the fence, on the lower slopes of the mountain, was a cluster of broken down shacks with dogs, children and big old wrecked cars. I had seen the people from here hanging around the shopping mall in town, smoking, sometimes drunk, generally aimless. Our neighbours complained they were not worth employing, being 'lazy and unreliable'. I looked at the mountain. They can't have been lazy or unreliable to survive in this landscape before the *'Canajians'* came and unilaterally rearranged the way people lived here.

Tzuhalem was everything our life was not, everything I came here to get away from. The shacks were the vicarage, the cars the wrecks that Pete endlessly did up in the yard outside. I was where I wanted to be in the nice, neat little VW – but my throat was constricted with longing because of that derelict, depressing, drug-laden scene.

'Stop a minute,' I said.

'What, here?'

'Yes, here.'

'But it's awful,' Hannah protested. She pulled the car into the side of the road.

'It's awful what they've done to these people. Taken away their life and then accused them of being idle and drunk.'

Hannah turned off the engine and sighed. 'You're always so taken up with what is going on in the world,' she complained. 'It's nothing to do with us.

I got out of the car, persuaded her to follow me and took her arm.

'Look. Look at those cars. Pete had cars just like that parked outside Hugh and Deidre's house. He was always working on them and never finished.'

Hannah pulled her arm away, irritated. 'That family of yours. Can't you ever just leave them alone?'

I was angry. 'I *have* left them alone. I've come six thousand miles away from them. I'm just saying it reminds me, that's all.'

We got back in the car and drove on, but it was the beginning of a slow, unstoppable alienation. I did not belong in our ordered life, and I began to resent Hannah and her family for being so at home in it. We lived surrounded by great natural beauty but we were long way from any big cities, and I also missed the things that Corinna had introduced me to – art, theatre, good music. I missed sophistication. I was tired of having to explain myself every time I made a joke. As time went on I longed more and more for England.

Hannah was restless in a different way. She missed male sex and her biological clock was running out. She longed for children while I was secretly relieved that we could not have them. In this I reminded myself of my father. When I was three, my mother had suffered a miscarriage at about three months: the baby was a boy. Having seen my father's look of relief when I told him Nana was dead, I was convinced that he was also secretly relieved not to have any more children.

Hannah and I needed each other, but we also loved each other enough to break up before the relationship became destructive. She drove me to the airport, where we held each other and wept before I went through to Departures. Her body was so familiar, but already it belonged somewhere else.

England was cramped, dirty and expensive but it was a relief to be back. I could not face London after the quiet of the West coast and settled in a provincial city where Jane, one of my university friends, already lived. It had plenty going on but it was also easy to escape into the countryside. You could engage in repartee without people looking blank. I rented a flat in a converted stone cottage in the old part of town. Mine was the bay window with deep windowsills and tasteful ornaments – the kind of window I had gazed into with longing as a child. Even without Hannah I found I could order my own home. Jane, now married and pregnant, was enjoying her own domestic scene alongside a part time social work job. I began to think that marriage, babies and being a woman was not all bad, and she even got me interested in clothes and sewing.

Meanwhile, I had no idea what to do next, and my savings would not last for ever. I had references from my teaching job and experience of social work, but no qualifications. While I thought about applying for – and funding – courses, I cast around for a job. One Saturday morning I noticed an ad in the local paper for a female graduate to work in a small graphic design company as a general assistant (this was before the Sex Discrimination Act). The pay was not bad, so I applied.

I fell in love with a voice on the telephone that invited me for an interview.

It was summer and I wore a dress I had made myself from a pink Laura Ashley fabric with little white flowers.

Jim Shaw in the flesh was nothing like his voice. The voice had worn a dark suit and sat behind a large polished desk in a calm, spacious office. Jim ran his business from a sprawling Victorian house near the canal, where he also lived. I pushed open the unlocked door and walked in.

For years afterwards I was to ask myself what happened when I stepped into that room. It was lined with makeshift shelves covered with papers in untidy heaps. Although there were built in desks against all the walls, there were no clear surfaces. Amongst the heaps of forms and letters were a couple of typewriters, an electronic composer and a telephone. A huge plastic dustbin overflowed with scrunched up paper, torn envelopes, filthy rags, teabags and dead flowers. In one corner was a kettle surrounded by used mugs, jugs and jars. Except that it was an office, it was my mother's kitchen. What happened? Instead of walking straight out again I stepped into that room as though into a warm bath. It was Tzuhalem all over again, only this time there was no wire fence to keep me out.

Jim sat in the midst of his chaos on a swivel chair, wearing an open necked shirt with the sleeves rolled up, and cotton trousers. He was in his late forties, with long greying hair falling from a bald crown: you could say he had a tonsure. He did not get up when I walked in but swivelled round and asked what I wanted. When he realised I was there for an interview he seemed delighted, and gave me tea sweetened with grapefruit marmalade from a stone jar. He then introduced me to the two women designers working at drawing boards in the back room, and asked me what my foibles were. I couldn't think of any but he was impressed that I had made my own dress, and the interview continued over a glass of white port. Two days later I received a postcard offering me the job and I took it.

The business produced designs for booklets, posters, advertisements, calendars and so on. Jim was not himself an artist, but he knew how to employ them and help them develop a house style that worked. Although he was a bit overweight he was vigorous and fit, and had spent time after the Second World War in army officer training, from which he had an endless fund of funny stories. From time to time, working in a different part of the house, I would hear shouting and go to investigate what was going on. More often than not it was Jim doing his impression of a sergeant major.

Before the army, by a strange coincidence, he had been at the same school as my father, and although he arrived some years later he described the same barbarous regime: 'The food was terrible: great slops from a pot, and if anyone ever enquired what it was the only reply was "Don't ask"'. 'The tuck shop was essential to survival. At least you could buy Ovaltine there to have with your bread and marge at tea – the jam was so bad that no-one could eat it …' 'We were glad when it snowed – because the pipes froze and no-one could force us to have a cold shower.'

42

Whereas my father had talked about the place with a certain pride and acceptance, Jim's only reaction was outrage. His eyes bulged and he thumped the desk whenever he talked about schools of any kind. I was excited by his capacity to get very angry indeed (he was renowned for paying difficult customers to go away). He appeared not to have heard of guilt, except in other people, and this, too, I found refreshing.

Working for Jim was fun. All kinds of people were in and out of the office, and my job was to keep tabs on everything – the admin, accounts, invoicing, marketing, and buying sandwiches at lunch time. The designers were delighted to have someone willing to take these things in hand, and although it was a gargantuan task, I enjoyed the infinite opportunities to make order out of chaos. The place buzzed with creativity, and was never boring. Above all, my job was free from guilt. If I messed up the worst that could happen was that a bill didn't get paid or someone didn't get their cup of tea. No-one needed my emotional help, and no-one would actually suffer if I failed to do something.

It was about a year before I ended up in Jim's bed. At Christmas I moved in with him, into his equally chaotic bedroom above the business, sharing a kitchen and bathroom with the various students who rented the other rooms. My beautiful flat lay discarded and empty. I was in love with a man nearly twenty years older than I was. To my amazement I also found I was desperate for a child.

If I was going to love a man, you could at least say that Jim was as different from Corinna as anyone could ever hope to be. And Jim was not remotely religious. He bitterly resented the number of services he had been forced to attend in the school chapel: twice a day for five years. His only religious phase had been in his late twenties, when, realising that he did not believe anything he had been taught, he became afraid of being condemned to hell. He dealt with this by going around repeating to himself incessantly, 'God is not a bloody fool' in the hope that this would protect him from blaspheming. Before long he realised this was a waste of effort, and he never worried about it again.

I took Jim to be the antithesis of my father, failing to take in that physically I could barely tell them apart: when they were in the same room I was simply aware of two round and balding men. My father only once expressed an opinion. It was after Jim mowed my parents' lawn for them, and he remarked, 'Someone who mows your lawn can't be all bad.'

My mother, however, was more than ready to express their views on my living with Jim. His age did not bother them. After all, my mother said, Nana's husband had been much older than she was (blithely ignoring the fact that he was hardly a shining example of an uxurious husband). My parents' problem, as communicated by my mother, was that I was 'living in sin'. Although Jim and I lived miles from their parish in another place altogether, she constantly complained that this was an embarrassment for my father. 'Why don't you just go ahead and get married', she suggested, 'It is so difficult for your father, and divorce is so easy these days if it goes wrong.'

When Jim and I did get married, we had a quiet Registry Office wedding, to which I reluctantly invited my parents a week before it took place. I was three months pregnant. The witnesses were Jane, pregnant again and accompanied by her two year old son, and Franny, my other best friend from Oxford. We could not have had a church wedding since Jim had been divorced some years before, but I refused to let my father perform any kind of service of blessing.

Kathy was born the following February, on the anniversary of Nana's death. The coincidence stirred in me a sense of something being set right by this new association with that sad date, but my mother was upset, as though I had been tactless in my timing.

It was Jim, much to my surprise, who suggested we get my father to baptise the baby. This had not occurred to me, but I contacted the local vicar to ask if we could use his church for the service. I wondered if we were supposed to pay him a fee, and at the end of our conversation I asked, 'Is there anything we should do about you?'

'You could try coming to church occasionally,' he replied. He had to be joking. I put the phone down, but by then I was able to pass on the arrangements to my father and it went ahead.

Back in their own parish – the same one I had left years before – my parents had got themselves involved in web of lies that made visiting them with Kathy embarrassing until she was of an age that was measured in years rather than months. I should perhaps have realised what was going on because when I sent out the birth announcements my mother rang almost straight away.

'How could you send Aunt Ede a birth announce-ment?' she demanded. I was bewildered. Aunt Ede was the only great-aunt who still happened to be alive: I thought it had been rather good of me to remember to send her one.

'What do you mean?'

'She didn't know you were already expecting when you got married.'

Worse was to follow. When Kathy was three months old, I got a sudden rush of birth congratulation cards from members of my father's parish. It was then that I realised they had only just now been told about her.

'They ask when she was born,' my mother was fond of saying, 'and I tell them she was born during the Sunday night Muppet Show', adding triumphantly, 'which is absolutely true.'

Shortly after those cards arrived I had a dream:

I come downstairs in the morning and find a lot of envelopes fallen through my letterbox. When I open them they contain black edged cards on which is written, 'Congratulations on the death of your baby.'

All this made me angry, but none of it struck me as strange. It was because it was like this that I had put church and everything to do with it well behind me. I just did not have to live like that anymore.

In another way, too, I had crossed a bridge. Married to Jim I found that I no longer identified with my father. Being Jim's wife was not always easy, but I loved him, and becoming a mother seemed to me an extraordinary and marvellous achievement. I took to it, though it did not occur to me until much later that I might get away – as I thought of it – with having more children.

4

Death and Discovery

EACH MORNING I dropped Kathy off at her nursery school and worked in Jim's office until it was time to pick her up. One day they phoned to say she was ill and needed to be collected early. I dropped everything and hurried to the school, and there she was sitting in a big arm chair in her little navy blue tracksuit, looking pale and tired. When she saw me walk in her face lit up. It was a life changing moment: she really wanted me, and it was all right that she should really want her mother when she didn't feel well – and I was there. It was overwhelmingly benevolent, and I could hardly bear it.

The following April, when Kathy had just turned four, my parents came to stay in a nearby bed and breakfast for a week and looked after her while I was working. I organised things for them to do each day, and cooked for us all in the evenings. On the last night I roasted a chicken for supper, and put the left overs in the fridge before Jim, Kathy and I went to Holland for a long weekend. We saw the sights of Amsterdam, and visited bulb fields with tulips taller than Kathy, Edam where the cheese comes from, and the model city at Madurodam. Then we caught the night boat back, and drove home. Jim dived into the office and

Kathy and I went upstairs to our living room. As I walked in the phone was ringing. I picked it up, and it was my brother Pete. 'Are you sitting down?' he asked.

'No.'

'Well, I think you'd better.'

'Why?'

'Hugh died last night.'

It had been a normal evening – for them. Hugh had disappeared into his study and written a sermon about the road to Emmaus, which ended 'Shall not our hearts, too, burn within us when we meet the risen Lord?' Deidre played the piano a bit and when he emerged he sat beside her and tinkled on the upper keys. Then he went to bed. She stayed up as she always did, and at around four she took up his breakfast: a slice of ham, bread and butter and a flask of tea. She always did this so that he could have breakfast in bed in the morning without disturbing her (no longer did he have an early daily Mass). She walked into their bedroom with the tray, and he was lying in his usual place on his side of their big wooden double bed.

Only he was dead.

Pete said that he had woken up around four: he had a strong sense that Hugh was in the room saying goodbye – and then the phone rang and it was Deidre. He went immediately to the vicarage, brought the breakfast tray down and threw the ham in the bin. 'That was a good slice of ham,' Deidre protested.

I had been on the boat when Hugh died and no presence had dropped by to say goodbye to me, which upset me a lot. I had always expected to know when he died, and I felt left out, ignored.

That night I got the cold chicken out of our fridge. 'I can't believe', I said to Jim, 'that a few days ago he was sitting here eating chicken.'

'Same chicken', replied Jim grimly.

I arranged for Kathy to stay with Jane's family, and went to London for three days. My aunt Cordelia joined us there too. We drove Deidre around from place to place – registry office, undertakers, florists – while she babbled incessantly. She was chain smoking which was odd since she was not a smoker: perhaps she wanted the smell of Hugh's cigarettes. She stunned us by insisting that we should wear hats for the funeral, so Cordelia and I went out and bought hats, giggling like naughty school girls.

Hugh was embalmed and brought back in his vestments to his study, where he lay in an open coffin so that people could come and make their farewells. His face looked spongey and lopsided, like a *Spitting Image* caricature of himself. I concentrated on the tips of his ears, which were slightly purple the way they always were.

The funeral was at the same church where I had once been organist. This was the first family funeral where I did not play the organ (Deidre was a bit upset when I declined), so there was no hiding in the organ loft. Pete refused to serve, as well. This was our father. It was up to other people to make the service happen. It did not work. Pete and I were once more the vicarage children on show in the front pew, maintaining a stiff upper lip in the presence of the coffin. Neither of us cried.

The funeral was taken by the local bishop, and began with a Eucharist celebrated by several of Hugh's colleagues. In his sermon the bishop said it was appropriate that we should be 'gathered round the table that Hugh loved'. I'd never thought of my father *loving* the Eucharist. It was simply something that he did. Did the bishop know things about him that I didn't? Was that the secret of my father – where he really had been all those years?

After the service, my mother could not stop talking, and the more she talked the more I withdrew into myself. She turned to Pete and said, 'She always did clam up like that when she was upset.'

At the burial Deidre nearly fell in the grave and had to be lifted away from the edge. Then, as we left the church-yard, a nun came up to Jim and me, peered up into his face and said, 'I know who you are – you're the new Father Nash.'

Jim thoroughly enjoyed the wake because it was full of Hugh's old friends from school. For the first time ever, he got to talk with other ex-pupils about how dreadful it all was. Then it was all, horribly, over, and we could go home.

In spite of the church funeral, it never occurred to me to talk to Kathy – who was experiencing death for the first time – about any kind of afterlife. It was not that I was against the idea. I longed for some way to explain to her what had happened to Grandpa, but I was at a loss. Grandpa had seemed perfectly OK when we had seen him and now he was dead. What was 'dead'? We gazed sadly at a dead goose on the river bank: that was 'dead' all right, but why should this happen, and how do you deal with it? It was only a few days after the funeral, when Kathy and I were playing together with her toy farm, that I had a sudden thought. 'Some people ...' I suggested hesitantly, 'believe that when you die you go to heaven.'

'What's heaven?'

'Well, it's a place where everything is perfect and everyone is happy, and you meet up with all your old friends again.'

Kathy immediately turned away from the farm and began playing with two of her stuffed toys as Grandpa meeting an old friend in heaven.

I was shocked that I had not thought of that before.

Before the funeral, while he lay there in the coffin in his vestments, I had investigated Hugh's study thoroughly. I felt entitled: at last he was going to tell me who he was, even if he had not said goodbye to me. In his desk drawer was the small Letts diary that he had bought to record anniversaries when he was ordained in 1944. Whenever a parishioner or a relative died he wrote their name and the year on the relevant page so he could remember them at Mass. I looked to see who else had died on 18 April, but there was a misprint – there was no 18 April in that diary. I hastily returned it to the drawer.

There were his journals that recorded next to nothing: the events of a particular day, where he'd been, who he had seen, but no clues as to how he felt about any of it – even when something concerned me. The saddest parts were his annual resolutions for observing Lent: no marmalade at breakfast; no alcohol at lunchtime …. I slipped one of them in my bag, hoping that there might be something there if I looked hard enough later on.

Among his books, however, there was one whose title attracted me because it was also the title of a Noel Coward song: *Some Day I'll Find You*. I took it, and when I finally got around to reading it, it turned out to be the autobiography of Harry Williams, a monk who had once been a Cambridge college chaplain, who was gay, and who had a breakdown over his love for a younger man. After that he went into psychoanalysis and finally decided he was called to be a monk. Having realised that, he hoped against hope that it might not happen. He developed a rash all over his body and promised himself that if it spread to parts that were visible outside his cassock he could abandon the monastic calling. The rash went neatly as far as his wrists, and stopped. So there he was in the monastery.

Harry Williams was gloriously ambivalent about church. For example, my father had railed against the new *versus populum* style of celebrating Mass – facing the people – but Harry Williams embraced it with relief. No longer would he have to stand with his back to the congregation, fighting the dread that someone was going to creep up on him.

Maybe in a church that had room for Harry Williams, there was room for me. I wrote to him and he replied, and I started to pray. The TV film *Shadowlands*, the story of C.S. Lewis and Joy Davidman, was released about this time. Moved by the film, I read Lewis's *A Grief Observed*. The way Lewis was prepared to challenge his own beliefs and their implications for the woman he loved was marvellous. Did I think my father had gone to heaven? I certainly did not think he had vanished into any kind of void. He was around, he was in my dreams, but he was also in my waking mind. We talked as we had never talked before. I felt I might be beginning to get close to him at last. But I could not find him in the churches.

5

Doing the Rounds

FOR THE FIRST TIME IN MY LIFE I had a friend who was a churchgoer. Annie ran a nursery where Kathy went on the mornings when I was working. She had a small tribe of her own children and Kathy loved them. Annie and I instantly liked each other and it was intriguing to discover that she was a member of the local church. Here was a true novelty: someone who was both religious and a natural friend for me. I began to wonder if I had lost something by not going to church all this time, and Annie invited me to an Easter Vigil – a service I remembered from my teens as mysterious and exciting. The reality was disappointing. Yes, it was the same service, but it was not my father taking it, and I left in tears. At Christmas I took Kathy to a carol service at a different church but she hated it. It was her first experience of pews and all that went with them, and I realised that nothing else in her life was anything like this.

It occurred to me, though, that I missed playing the organ, and from time to time, leaving Kathy with Jim, I filled in at a non-conformist church which I liked because the people seemed gentle and sincere. Everyone was over fifty, except for one family who had one child. He was a very good child, and always sat quietly in the front row. These people heard the Word of God, and apparently kept it, and were involved in various good works. They all knew how to sing, and they sat and listened politely at the end until I had finished the organ voluntary.

One Sunday, the minister was not there and someone told me that his wife had died suddenly. Horrified for him, I wrote him a letter of sympathy. He wrote back and invited me to visit him at his house, where he gave me a cup of tea and told me how he hated the things people said about his wife's death. He particularly hated the cards which said 'Death is nothing at all'. 'Death is everything' he said.

Next time I went to play at the church they told me he was on extended sick leave. His replacement was a woman and for me this was another revelation – a woman presiding in church. Some Sundays she would celebrate communion and extemporise on the prayers:

'We break your body, and your body is torn, as Mary's body was torn when she gave birth.' *Hey.* The congregation seemed to take her along with everything else in their stride. No-one walked out. They seemed to appreciate her for what she was. I certainly did.

One evening I rang the regular minister again to see how he was, and he was drowning in grief. He took to ringing me up, and I was touched by the way he confided in me. Then, late one evening, I heard in his voice the note of alcoholic self-pity familiar to me from drinkers around my mother's kitchen table. The next time I went to the church, they told me he was dead. 'Poor John,' they said. 'The grief was simply too much for him.' I had never met people as good as this. So what did I do? I stopped going there. I could not take such goodness.

My next experiment was with a convent, which reminded me of the first book Corinna ever lent me, Iris Murdoch's *The Bell*. Although I entered by invitation into the guest chapel, I felt all the terror of trespass that Dora does when she climbs into the convent over the wall, and received all the same impervious kindness. Before long, I started going there regularly for a weekday Eucharist. It was marvellous to me that they had kept all this going while I had been away from it, and that they shared it so generously.

The Eucharist was simple, and I loved it. We, the guests, sat in a section at right angles to the sanctuary, and never saw the chapel itself – just the nuns when they came up to communion. But you knew that day and night someone prayed in there. You could feel it welcoming and enfolding you the moment you opened the door. At any time you could come and pray with them, and you never had to know anything about them, or they anything about you. There were all the benefits of liturgy without any of the social trappings. It was perfect.

One day I parked my car and headed towards the chapel as usual. As I opened the door to the antechapel I found myself confronted by all the nuns processing out. The nun leading them looked startled and I fell back, but someone gestured to me to follow them to another building, which it turned out they were using temporarily while the chapel was being painted. It was a simple enough mistake – there was no reason why I should have known about this. But though I managed to get through the service I was devastated. I felt myself to be some kind of monstrous being who had burst in and trampled on holy ground. It went with an overwhelming sense of shame. When I got back in the car I had a major panic attack.

Although the nuns were contemplatives, they began to move with the times and became a bit more outgoing. Someone gave them an electronic organ, and guests were brought into the main chapel. They had hymns instead of their beautiful quavery unaccompanied plainsong. The hymns made me cry. I stopped going so regularly and started looking around at other possibilities.

Briefly, I played the organ at an evangelical church and enjoyed the rumbustious singing – until it suddenly filled me with despair. I could not detect anything underneath the melodies. Then there was the way that people seemed strung out with the effort of preserving their bounce and stretching their lips in a smile. One woman had the habit of saying 'How are you?' while simultaneously smiling and shutting her eyes. When I found myself wanting to hit her, hard, I decided it was time to move on.

The best churches, I decided, were empty ones. One day when I had dropped off Kathy at a friend's house in a nearby village, I went into the village church. It was quiet, and I settled myself in the choir stalls, huddled up against the pulpit, and shut my eyes, feeling safe and enclosed. Even when I heard some high heels come clacking in, I stayed put with my eyes shut. Whoever it was would go away when they had done whatever they had come for. The sound came closer and I thought maybe they had some business in the sanctuary. Then, unmistakably, the heels started to advance down my choir stall and a body settled itself beside me. I had noticed this about churches. Even when there was a service you could go into an almost empty church, select a nice quiet position as far as possible from anyone else – and the next person to come in would come and sit right beside you.

Now, however, there was not even a service going on. And this person was not just sitting beside me, but staring at me. I could feel it through my eyelids. Which gave way to the pressure, and opened on a pair of intense brown eyes.

It was some woman to do with the church, a warden, maybe. 'Hallo' she said.

My look clearly failed to convey my feelings since she did not shrivel into ashes. Instead she announced she was a deaconess and asked if I was all right.

'Yes, thank you, 'I said, 'I just came in here to pray.'

Still she did not take the hint.

'Beautiful church, isn't it,' she said.

'Yes.'

'And where do you normally worship?'

Outrage gave way to panic. The question flooded me with vicarage guilt, and I was simply incapable, for some reason, of saying 'Nowhere'. 'So sorry, I have to go now,' I said, and pushed past her out of the church.

All the same, my researches turned up a good many people who seemed to me something extraordinary – sincere, gentle, good people, who prayed and lived trustworthy lives. The trouble was, I could not bear being near them – not because of them, but because of me. However hard I tried, I could not be with them and also be myself. I would become polite, and smile, and tell them what an interesting and fulfilling life I had, what a nice husband and what a lovely daughter, what satisfying work...

I had learned something though. I had learned that prayer was tangible, so I kept to that in the privacy of my own home, as best I could. It was lonely, praying alone, and hard to get an idea of what I was supposed to be doing. I knew prayer when I recognised it, but I was not sure how to find it except by a sort of listening inside myself. Sometimes I found a sense of a loving God. At other times a cocktail of guilt and anger. The figure of Christ bothered me a lot. Hanging there on his cross he seemed manipulative, reproachful: *Look how you've made me suffer*. My response was rage. I wanted to be there on Golgotha and hammer in the nails myself.

The look of reproach reminded me of my mother, now living in a little terraced house stuffed with the contents of a fifteen room vicarage, with no expansive kitchen to invite people into. How could I sit there praying for her, when sixty miles away she was drinking her way through lonely evenings? I really should go and see her more often. The next Saturday, I left Jim at the office and set off with Kathy for a visit.

'What does "Hour of our death" mean' asked Kathy as we got in the car.

'Well, it's the moment when you die'

'What?' said Kathy.

'It's from the Hail Mary. "Hail Mary, full of grace the Lord is with thee. Blessed art thou among women and blessed is the fruit of thy womb, Jesus. Holy Mary, Mother of God, pray for us sinners now and at the hour of our death ." '

The Angelus. Perkins on the bell rope. Me standing beside him, looking up at him as he muttered the words, watching him make the bell of St George's ring out to remind everyone it was twelve noon, time to pray. Three, three, three, then nine. And the 'Hail

Mary's' in between.

I felt quite smug about having this piece of Christian heritage to pass on to my daughter.

'Mum, are you all right?'

'Sure.'

'But Mum, I wanted to know what that knob was for – the one that says "RR DEF"'

'Oh.' *Oh?*

'It's the rear screen defrost – heats up the back window when it's misted up'

'Fine,' said Kathy. 'Shall we put a tape on?'

As well as praying I read a lot, grazing at random in the Bible where I found the song of Hannah, the story of Sarah and Abraham, Isaiah, the Song of Songs, the psalms. All these seemed much more interesting than the New Testament. It occurred to me that I had no real idea what Christianity was about, and with that went a sense that praying alone was not enough. Eventually, I asked Annie, who knew everyone and most things about them, if she had any good ideas as to what might work for me.

'You could if you wanted,' she said, 'go and have a chat with Father Richard. He's a man of prayer and he knows his way around. I don't suppose he'd mind.' Annie was always right about people, so if she said this Father Richard would not mind, I could count on it he would not.

Accordingly, one Monday I rang him. I knew he would not be there because my father had always had Mondays off – and he wasn't. A few weeks later I rang again, on a Tuesday, and told him Annie had given me his number.

'Would you like to come round?' he asked.

'Yes,' I said, reaching for my door-keys.

'Let's see if we can arrange a time then.'

'Of course.' I put the keys down.

A few days later there I was, on the unfamiliar side of a vicarage door. I rang the bell and Father Richard answered. By now I knew he was married with teenage children, and in his fifties. He was tall and slim, and fitted neatly into a dark clerical suit which showed no traces of egg yolk or tobacco ash. He had nice eyes.

He invited me into his study, which felt calm and safe, not tidy or untidy, but as though it lived with him in a relationship of amiable neglect. I just managed to stop myself from making the sign of the cross as I walked in. We sat down in shabby but comfortable armchairs placed at an angle so we were not quite facing each other. He smiled. I noticed he was not the other side of a desk. I hoped he could not see that I was shaking. As for him, he sat there as though he had all the time in the world. I plunged in. 'I've never done this before, sat down with a priest I mean. My father was one, you see.'

He smiled again, so I told him what I had always longed to tell my father, how I had left the Church because I could not be with Corinna and stay in it. His listening was quiet, and very relaxed. When I finished, there was a pause. Then he said the last thing on earth I expected him to say.

'You did the right thing.'

'I did?'

'You see,' he said, 'you had reached a point where you wanted two things that for you were incompatible. You realised you had to make a choice – so you made one.'

'But I walked away from God.'

'I shouldn't worry about that,' he said. 'After all, God was not going anywhere.'

'But I chose her over communion.'

'Well,' he said, 'I can see that it might have been difficult for you to go to communion in the circumstances. Maybe it was better to stay away. But there are many different ways of belonging to a church. If it were one of my own children, I think I'd be inclined to say – yes – I think I'd say hold off communion for the time being, but you are always welcome in church.'

He would, would he? Was it possible that a father could ever speak to his children like that? One thing that was extraordinary about Father Richard was that he did not even seem very interested in my story. He gave the impression he'd seen it all before – not that he did not care, but the story was not the most interesting thing. It was the problem that was interesting.

A few months later, I went to a Sunday morning service at his church, the same one where Annie had taken me to the Easter vigil the year before. It looked different in daylight, with the sun streaming in, lighting up the columns of incense smoke. All the trappings of St George's were there: candles, a rood screen with statues of the Apostles – though the altar was in front of it. There was a pulpit, but it was full of plants and obviously never used for preaching. There was a wooden statue of Mary and Jesus, but she was neither holding him up like a little potentate nor absorbed in maternal tenderness. She was holding him out head first towards the people, his arms outstretched and her hand supporting him underneath as though she was teaching him to swim. Loving him and letting go. I was to spend many hours staring at that statue. Near the altar two Orthodox icons hung on the screen, of Christ and Mary. That day I barely noticed them, but they, too, were to become part of my inner landscape.

The organist was playing Bach chorales I knew almost by heart: *Liebster Jesu, wir sind hier*; *Schmücke dich, o liebe Seele...* I felt glad to know them. They did not hurt. My gentle re-acquaintance with the organ had worked.

At communion everyone went up to the rail while I sat in an agony of indecision. I had had breakfast before I came though I knew from my aunt Cordelia that the fast was only an hour now, not from midnight, and it was well past that by now. The services at the convent were so early that I had never thought about that, but simply went straight there after getting up and had breakfast when I got home. Here everything felt different. I did not know if I belonged or not – or wanted to. *Love bade me welcome but my soul drew back ...*

Even so, I realised that I had come home, and from then on I went every week, listening as though my life depended on it to every word of the services. Each time we said the Creed I would be asking myself, *Do I believe that or not? what difference does it make?* I could never forget the martyrs who were tortured and died – and were still being tortured and dying in some parts of the world – for this story. I had always wondered whether I would believe in Christianity if it were forbidden. Why were the lives of the saints always so grim? Then there was the Lord's Prayer: *what did it mean to say, 'Your Kingdom come'? What was this kingdom? And did I actually desire it?*

When, after a few weeks, Annie persuaded me to stay for church coffee, I found there were other people asking themselves these kinds of questions and what they meant to them in everyday life. It was a thriving, cosmopolitan congregation in the heart of town – a far cry from the suburbia of my father's parish. It was also quite different from the family style of belonging to church. When I was growing up the church was our life, but none of the people at St George's were quite real. Hugh gave them nicknames: my first recollection of death was him coming into the sitting room and announcing 'Eagle Wings has grown his wings.' Both he and Pete were expert mimics and story tellers. We did not expect to enter into the world of the parishioners, nor them into ours.

Father Richard and his family did not seem to behave like that. There was continuity between them and their role in the church. And for the first time, church was a place where I could be myself: there was Annie, and there were other people I would have been glad to know as friends even if church did not exist. All my life I had assumed it was only a matter of time before the church died, but these people seemed to think it was very much alive.

I went to all the discussion groups and talks that I could. It also turned out that Richard (I soon dropped the 'Father') was a scholarly man, and from him, too, I learned a great deal. He always seemed happy to talk about Trinity and Incarnation, and about the Eucharist.

It was several months before I felt ready to receive communion, and he was entirely relaxed about this, encouraging me to take my time. I got the impression he did not want me to do anything in a hurry. There were many ways, he said, to participate in the Eucharist, just as there were many ways of belonging to church.

The first time I did go up to the rail and receive the bread and the wine was not on a Sunday but just after Christmas at a quiet weekday Mass for the 'Holy Innocents' – the children slaughtered by Herod when he heard that the Messiah had been born. It was still dark outside. Annie was there, and just a few other people. She knew that this was the day I was going to receive communion there for the first time and had brought me a small book of Celtic poetry which she gave me after the service. *You must sit down, said Love, and taste my meat. So I did sit and eat.*

I had no recollection of communion meaning anything when I was a child except as a duty you had to perform every Sunday. Now it became an essential part of my weekly rhythm, and as my therapy practice developed it nourished me. Whatever happened during the week, I was immersed in something entirely different on Sunday morning. It gave me a sense of oneness, not just with the congregation that day, but also with people everywhere, and with people who had died. Even more important was being accepted, being allowed to take part, being given the bread and wine, the body and blood of Christ. It was a human sharing, but it was also a gift that told me I was loved. Even the words began to sound different. 'This is my body ... This is my blood'. When the Christ in the icon on the rood screen spoke these words they did not feel reproachful. I began to hear them as the love of a cosmic Christ, not one who insisted on being victimised, but one who suffused the whole of creation. *This* – the simple staple food – *is my body; the wine is my blood. Eat. Drink. Remember me.*

As for Mary, Annie and I had many conversations about her, because I was intrigued by the other icon on the screen. She looked nothing like the skimpy statues of my youth – 'Nothing between the hip bones' as Annie put it. She explained to me that Mary, too, was identified with creation and that her feasts followed the rhythm of nature. She was taken up into heaven as the harvest was brought in, and conceived as the first seeds were sown in the ground. I loved living in the annual rhythm of liturgical feasts. They spoke of life, death and resurrection – birth in the darkness of winter, death giving way to new life in the spring, the falling away of the old year as summer gave way to autumn. They spoke of continuity and I was part of it.

By this time I had learned not to volunteer to get involved in the music. I had no desire to take up the organ again, and I kept away from the choir. I was relishing being simply part of something without responsibilities. I loved the church, the liturgy, the community. What I did not realise was that there was a powerful reaction to it all going on deep inside me. Shortly after I began going once more to communion, I had a dream:

Jim, Kathy and I are staying in a large old house with a slightly mad couple in charge, next door to an abbey where the nuns are also a little mad – tuned in to a way of life that does not fit with the here and now.

Our host, a retired colonel, over a very good dinner, tells us the legend of the abbey. At one time, around a hundred years earlier, the nuns went in for infanticide at Easter. As part of the ceremony they hung up a special symbol of three interlocking circles.

Kathy goes to bed, and the rest of us are drinking, and Jim gets very drunk indeed. Then someone comes in and says how marvellous it is that the nuns still keep to the old customs. They have just been across to the abbey, and there, hung up, was the sign of the three overlapping circles.

Immediately I know what this means: that is the sign they hang up when they have killed a child, and I also know that child is Kathy.

I woke from this dream – and woke Jim – shouting, 'They've killed her'. He went back to sleep but I went into another room to write the dream down. I was shaking, and it was hard to do. While I was writing, Jim came in because he thought I had been standing beside the bed saying his name to attract his attention. 'It was very powerful,' he said, 'not violent, but powerful. I've never known anything like it, and I don't like it.'

It was another year before I dreamed of St George's:

I am trying to get into St George's through the back door. I seem to be running away from something. I have a key and get in, and a black dog comes up behind me. I hastily shut the door to keep him out, but it doesn't seem right and I can't lock the door from inside. Each time I think I've done it and push the door to check, it falls open. The dog ends up on my side of the door, in the role of a companion. Meanwhile the lock transforms into a sexual image, and I have to work to get something the shape of a penis into the right hole. I can't do it and I call for help.

By this time I was in therapy, but we had much else to talk about, and I did not take these churchy dreams there. Also, the black dog of depression was far away. It would be several years before I would discover him to be my companion – even, eventually, my friend.

Part 2
THERAPY

Once, stretched out on her lap
as now on a dead tree,
I learned to make her smile,
to stem her tears,
to undo her guilt,
to cure her inward death.
To enliven her was my living.

Donald Winnicott

1

The Glass Butterfly

IF MY ADULT RELATIONSHIP with church began with the death of my father, my career in therapy began with threatening to kill my mother. I never did learn what Winnicott learned – to enliven her.

For as long as I could remember, my relationship with my mother was suffused with anxiety and a vague sense of dread. All her conscious intentions were generous and loving, she and my father were essential to each other, and she had some devoted friends, but for me she was pure pain. I was terrified of her – or rather of her effect on me.

Whatever she thought or felt seeped out of her into

anyone who had receivers on the appropriate wave length. Those who had adequate filters of their own were unaffected. For those who did not she was, as one person put it, 'pure poison'.

Being married to Jim gave me some protection against the creeping virus that was Deidre. If she wrote me a letter it smouldered on the doormat until I picked it up, and I always got Jim to open it and read it first. Jim was not completely immune, however, and once when I asked him what he thought about her, he replied, 'Everything she attaches herself to she slowly and steadily destroys.'

She did this in small but significant ways. Jim, for example, had the same name as my Uncle Jim who had been brain damaged at birth, and when we got married my mother said that we could not have two people in the family of the same name. This was especially senseless because being her, she never even called Uncle Jim 'Jim': it was always 'Jimmy' or 'Jamesie', and nobody else was going to get the two of them mixed up. Nevertheless, she tried to insist on everyone calling Jim by his middle name, Edward. I was livid – and there was no way Jim was suddenly going to change his name – but it was impossible to discuss our feelings about it with her. We simply ignored her when she called Jim 'Edward', and she eventually dropped it.

As for me I had no filters, and no-one had yet explained to me about maternal envy. For Jim's fiftieth birthday party, I bartered some graphic design work for a green silk designer dress. I had never worn anything like this before, and was amazed and enchanted by the sight of myself in the mirror. My mother arrived for the party, took one look and said, 'You do look nice. I think I'll go home.'

It was not intended to be malicious, and she stayed

for the party. But it was as though we could not thrive in in the same universe. I longed to make her happy, and having failed miserably I was consumed with guilt. Years after she died, I met a friend of Pete's who had spent a lot of time drinking whisky round her kitchen table. He reminisced at length, then unwittingly gave me his absolution.

'There was simply no room for a young woman in that house,' he said. 'Your father and Pete were like barons in their family seat, and Deidre became totally wife and mother. The only thing for you to do was to get out.'

For Pete it was different. While I never really lived at the vicarage after the affair with Corinna started, he stayed on until his late twenties, which was then unusual. Partly it was the alcohol – always freely available – that held him, and partly it was Deidre herself, and the power of her need for him. Even when he found a lifelong partner, Jeanine, and moved out he remained within her orbit, spending much of his time back at 'home'.

My murderous threat that took me into therapy was delivered around the same time that I began trying out churches. Deidre came to the pirate party I organised for Kathy's seventh birthday. I had stayed up half the night making a cake in the shape of a pirate galleon from *Children's Party Cooking*. Neither cake making nor modelling came naturally to me but the result was satisfying and the crew of piratical children cheered when I brought the cake in. They were enjoying themselves, and I felt happiness well up inside me that even with Deidre there, I was giving Kathy a good birthday. Then, during the games, something went wrong and Kathy started to cry.

'Don't cry on your birthday', said my mother.

The moment she said it I saw myself on my seventh birthday, standing on the garden path and crying because childhood was gone for ever. Instantly I knew what she was going to say next and my only thought was to stop her. She was the wicked witch cursing my child, and I spoke even as she said, 'If you cry on your birthday, you'll cry all year.'

What I had said was, 'If you say that, I'll kill you.'

It all passed so quickly that probably only I even noticed it, and the party went on. Later, however, I thought: *I threatened to kill my mother in front of a bunch of seven year olds. Perhaps I should try therapy.*

I duly referred myself to an NHS clinic, was offered an appointment and made my way to a quiet, bare waiting room in neutral colours. Just to sit there made me feel better. Then, to my dismay, a man walked in to collect me. It had never occurred to me that the therapist would not be a woman. It occurred to me to run away, but I had learned a thing or two working with Jim. *I am the consumer here*, I told myself – *just give it a try.*

Nevertheless I was a little scared of Mr O., a thin man in late middle age who wore a suit and tie. He was very quiet so you never knew what he was thinking, but whatever went on under that calm exterior was extremely attentive. On the rare occasions when he did speak it went straight to the point. After a couple of sessions, I was wondering if I really needed this, since I was already feeling better than I had done. He looked at me severely, and said, 'So you are feeling a bit better and want to stop?'

I felt rebuked for my shallowness, and decided to go on. Soon afterwards I had a vivid dream:

I am a little girl. There is a beautiful glass butterfly, a present from my father to my mother. By accident, I eat it, and as I feel the crunch of glass between my teeth, I become terrified that my insides are full of ground glass.

Mr O. and I worked with this dream as an image of how I had been affected by the miscarriage of my younger brother whom Deidre always referred to as Henry or 'that little one'. Though I had no direct memory of it – I was three when it happened – she had told me about it many times. It was the founding story of her depression, even down to the long brown coat she had that winter and the sense of despair that came over her every time she put it on.

It was a classic Deidre story of why you should never allow yourself to feel happy in case the Fates notice and destroy you. The first three months of her pregnancy had passed, and all through a Parish Council meeting in our dining room she hugged her secret inside her, quietly gloating over the dried up spinsters at the meeting; soon she could begin to tell people about the baby. That night, she suddenly went into labour, and was taken into hospital. While there she had to have her womb 'scraped out', and was told she could not have any more children.

According to Deidre the shape of my face changed in her absence, and became square. She also said that after she came home I used to help an invisible baby downstairs behind me, and once, when we were out shopping, I clapped my hand over my mouth and cried, 'We forgot the baby!'

It was also part of the story that Pete, who was seven at the time, developed alopecia and his hair fell out. She would tell us about these reactions with a kind of pride, as though both Pete and I had expressed the enormity of what had happened in a way that she could not.

Using my dream, Mr O. helped me explore the confusion in a small child's mind, and I began to form questions about what might have gone on for me at the time. Did I perhaps believe that I had destroyed the 'present' given by my father to my mother? Was it possible that I also believed I had fatally wounded myself – with ground glass – in the process?

The ground glass image was particularly appropriate. When I talked about Deidre it was as though there was something very tender inside me, like a sponge composed of raw nerve endings: if it were touched it would scream.

I had the same sensation when Kathy said to me one day that she had heard a song on the radio that reminded her of 'Didi'. Deidre had refused to be identified by any of the 'Grandmother' words: she did not want Kathy to think that she was old. 'Didi' was the best Kathy could do when she learned to speak, and it stuck. 'What was the song like?' I asked.

'It felt like an innocent child who thought everything was all right and didn't understand adult problems.'

Yes. This was both accurate and painful.

'How did it make you feel about her?' I asked.

'Please don't', she said. 'It's too awful.'

The raw thing inside me pulsated. Kathy, who had loved my mother when she was tiny, was repeating my own inability to continue to love Deidre as she grew up. At least she was experiencing this at the remove of one generation. It was still horrible, but she had some distance from it. Jim and I stood between her and Deidre.

When I began to explore the place of the miscarriage in my own psyche, I asked Pete, my brother, what he remembered, and he did not have to delve far to find his own memories.

'What I remember,' he said, 'is the sense of shock. Hugh coming into the room and telling me "Your mother's had to go into hospital", and thinking *Christ – it's happened to me*. I went to school in a state of shock. I was very calm – uneasily calm. I suppose that's why I got the alopecia. The doctor – she was Jewish – thought it was because there was a crucifix over my bed, but it wasn't. It was the shock.'

Pete's bald patch led to trouble with the verger's son, who often hung around the church garden in the school holidays.

'It looked a bit weird where my hair fell out and people used to go on about my Davey Crockett haircut. And there was Perks's son. I remember coming out of the vestry at the back of the church and him saying, "You've got a Davey Crockett haircut" and giving me a rabbit punch on the back of the neck and knocking me unconscious. Perks got severely told off, but I am sure that's why I hit him with a monkey wrench later on ...'

All this I knew, but then he said something astonishing. 'We went to visit her in hospital, and she wrote lots of letters, full of illustrations, which were magical.' Was Deidre a sort of E. Nesbit then? I had never thought of her that way. I had adored Nesbit's books as a child (though I later found her – as portrayed in a biography – irritating).

'Do you remember her coming home?' I asked.

'No,' Pete replied. 'I don't remember her coming home. Only that morning when she had gone into hospital and the sense of shock. Vividly. I dimly remember being psychologically prepared for a baby, and then there wasn't one. I remember Nana bustling about, but that's all.'

To me, it was a great deal. I had no idea whether I also had magical letters from the hospital, or was taken to visit. I was probably considered too young. It was typical that Pete remembered so much, and I nothing.

Whatever did happen that night, we were never allowed to forget the missing presence of Henry. It was as though there were three of us, but one just happened to be dead. I described to Mr O. how that very week I had said to Deidre at the end of a phone call, 'See you on Saturday.'

'I hope so,' she answered. 'I never dare look forward to anything since I lost that little one.'

Mr O.'s style was not to sympathise or interpret, but simply to comment on what he saw – or rather perceived in the strange still way he sat there. 'You're simply boiling with rage, aren't you,' he remarked, and I waited for the sky to fall because someone had noticed this. It did not.

With Mr O., I identified and managed to name the guilt, rejection and anxiety that went to make up the rage I felt against my mother and her depression. His comments were unfailingly accurate. One day towards the end of our time together he said, 'It seems as though you would like to bring your mother here and leave her here.'

Oh *yes*. That was exactly how I had felt all my life. If only she could be somewhere different, in the right place, she might be happy. It was marvellous to have someone recognise that.

Over a few months Mr O. succeeded in slowing me down in a way that made me feel taken seriously; he even managed to negotiate a few extra sessions for me because he thought I needed them. I was not sure whether to feel guilty or grateful about this.

It was during this 'extra' time that I had the panic attack at the convent when I felt as though I had violated the sanctuary. He listened carefully, and showed that he understood. Talking about it was terrifying – could I survive someone else hearing these thoughts of mine? – but amazingly, I found that I could indeed survive it.

When we came to our last session Mr O. said goodbye to me with words that were both infuriating and sustaining. 'After all,' he said, 'you are a going concern.' It was to be twelve years before I returned to discuss that comment with him.

2

Analysis

I CAME AWAY FROM MR O. with an important thought in my head: maybe there was no reason why I should not have a second – or even third – child just like anyone else. Until that point I had thought that I had done something so momentous, so against my own sense of what I was capable of, that I was lucky to get away with it. I discussed it with Jim and had my contraceptive coil removed. Almost immediately I got pregnant, but a few weeks later the baby miscarried. Not long afterwards Jim had a major emergency operation in which he nearly died. He recovered, but there was no possibility of more children. Almost crazy with grief, I went into therapy with a Jungian analyst, Patricia, who worked with me for five years.

Patricia was very different from Mr O. Whereas he was a small man, and his room at the clinic was quietly impersonal, Patricia was large and all embracing: her room over-flowed with welcome, and was lined with books, pictures and interesting objects. These were all part of the therapy. Staring at a shell, a beautiful stone, a painting of rolling hillsides, or even a row of books could be, I discovered, very soothing to one's inner thoughts. She was not the kind of analyst who puts you on a couch and waits for you to free associate: we sat in chairs opposite each other. Her quality of attention was different from Mr O.'s – she was much more interactive – but equally deep.

Early on, I had a dream whose significance only became clear years after we had finished our work together:

I have to go through some kind of initiation ceremony. There is a hooded, faceless figure who is the past and the future. Patricia is there as a guide, but she cannot come with me beyond this point. As she leaves, she writes me a huge cheque full of love and richness.

For the first few sessions, I wept a great deal, apologising profusely and being told that it was OK, I needed to get this out. Over the following months I learned that it was possible to have a miscarriage, and grieve – even bitterly – and recover. Again, my mother's miscarriage and how it had affected me was a major focus. It was a revelation to me when Patricia said, 'I can tell you that you were once devoted to your mother.'

The thought had never occurred to me. I assumed I had always been this dreadful ball of hatred and anxiety.

With Patricia's help I also rediscovered Nana, whom I had hardly thought about for years. Her death had been overlaid by the affair with – and loss of – Corinna. If I did refer to her, I said 'my grandmother'. To use the name of affection, 'Nana' was too painful, binding me to my mother's world in a way I could not bear. About a year into the analysis, however, I had what I called the 'grandmother cycle' of dreams:

1. Corinna is back in England and I have arranged to see her, but first I need to speak to her urgently, and I ring her up. 'You remember how much I grieved when my grandmother died?' I ask her.

'Yes'

'Then why is she suffering and dying now?'

Corinna answers, 'You know that sometimes these things have to be gone through in advance.'

2. My mother brings Nana to me and says, 'Look how dreadful this is. She's got Alzheimers. She can't even play the piano anymore.' I take Nana to the piano and she can play. It is not as good as in the past but it is good enough.

3. Beneath our house are large cellars that I have locked up. I discover that they have been opened, and are light and airy and full of old but good things Kathy has made. There, in the centre is the grandmother doll from my doll's house in perfect condition.

These dreams were very important to me. In the first, Corinna acts as a bridge to unresolved grief that was wiped out by what happened with her. Then I am able to reject my mother's doom laden verdict about Nana's state of mind (she never did suffer from dementia, though my mother used to complain that she was becoming 'childish' in her old age). Finally the third dream shows how the cellars of the mind that I have locked up are opening. This was the most important of the three dreams, and suggested to me that it was from Nana that I acquired what foundations for womanhood I had, that she had filled the space where my mother was missing, and that by becoming Kathy's mother I had somehow found her again. For the first time I realised that when Nana died it was like losing a mother. The devastation I felt then suddenly made sense.

There was now a chain of 'mothers': Nana, who had been secure but became ill and died; my own mother who had disappeared into depression and addiction; and then there was Corinna who had given me so much as a teacher but had used me as a lover and then abandoned me.

Patricia became the next in the chain. She was the first person to talk to me about love in a non-sexual way, and to be truly loving at the same time. She cherished me, but she also wanted me to grow up.

With her I revisited the affair with Corinna, who still remained my ideal to the extent that I was confused by the fact that I had got married and had a child – even though Kathy was the best thing that had ever happened to me. Finally, painfully, I came to accept that however much I loved her and valued all that she had opened up for me, what Corinna did was an abuse of her position. Patricia, an earth mother with three grown up children, became my new gold standard for womanhood. With her help I learned, painfully, to transform envy into gratitude, to learn from someone else while at the same time valuing myself.

Trusting Patricia did not come easily. Good parenting, it seemed, made me just as angry as bad parenting, and I resented her calmness, and her power. This did nothing to soften my desperate need of her. Neither with her nor with Mr O. did I discuss much childhood memory: I had very little of that. What I did have was deep wells of feeling that surfaced in the therapeutic process. The most prominent of these was separation anxiety. Often I simply did not know how to survive from one Wednesday to the next, and Patricia's three week summer holiday was agony. I dreaded these breaks, but I could not – as Patricia pointed out – bring myself to say, 'I don't want you to go'. She tried to get me to say it and I would not. I clung to her, but I did it in secret.

'What I have to get over,' I wrote in my journal as one of these breaks approached, 'is panic. Separation panic. It's not that I think she is going to die, or not come back. It's more that she's going to see her chance to get rid of me. That's why I secretly cling to her. It's like holding onto the underneath of the train so I don't get left behind.'

With Patricia I relived my feelings as a small child when my mother disappeared into depression. I also discovered inside myself what Patricia described as 'a miasmic black hole': a sense of total worthlessness into which I could tumble without any hope of rescue – except when I saw her. She eventually responded with a kind of irritation that I should project these feelings onto her, and this was bracing.

I also learned to rely on music, and in particular the slow movement of Shostakovich's second Piano Concerto. This has a gentle, lyrical melody which appears three times, and each time it comes back it is a simple joy to hear it again. The last time it comes, however, it is accompanied by some deep notes on the piano which tell you that this time you will have to say goodbye. I played this movement over and over again in the gaps between sessions. With Patricia's help I learned from it something about the difference between the separation that comes from growing up, and being 'untimely ripp'd'.

One day Patricia told me that her own mother had suffered badly from depression. 'When I was trying to cope with my own mother,' she said, 'I was working as a psychiatric social worker, and someone suggested that I write her up as a case. I found that very helpful. You've been a social worker. Why don't you try it?'

The idea appealed to me. Already I had begun to cope

with visiting my mother by thinking of it as a form of work, and now I imagined visiting her as a case worker. I 'wrote her up' in the format I had been taught as an assistant hospital social worker in the early 1970s.

Deidre Nash
Age 69
Family: Hd d. five years ago (occupation: vicar). 1 son, 1 daughter.

Presenting problems:
Depression. Tiredness. Difficulty managing housework / finances.

Health
History of tiredness and disturbed sleep patterns. Since 1960s dependent on amphetamines to 'keep going'. Also takes caffeine tablets to keep awake.
Complains of depression; lethargy; pains in feet and hip. Appetite poor, but not emaciated.

Cigarettes: none

Alcohol: 2-3 bottles of whisky per week.

Housing
Own 2-bedroomed house, poorly kept. Overstuffed with furniture and belongings; client does not go to bed because there is not room for her to get into it. Client complains of mess and of losing things. Refuses help in tidying house: 'I've parted with all I can bear to part with.'

Personal appearance

Client looks tired and depressed. Clothes clean but shabby – bits sewn on (lace cuffs etc) to lengthen sleeves, cover up neckline. Hair dyed and unkempt. Eyebrows twitch. Voice very flat.

Loss of husband

Hd died at home in bed after history of heart disease and diabetes. Client found him in bed when she went in with his breakfast. She had not been to bed herself. Blames herself that did not know how to resuscitate him. Also that she did not persuade him to have heart surgery, though he had said he would rather die than go through with it. ? resents his preference for death to staying with her ('He knew the children would be all right. He wasn't worried about leaving them. I don't know what he thought about leaving me.')

Practical implications of bereavement

Client had to a leave large vicarage for her present house which she bought with money hd put aside. Resents her reduced circumstances.
Blames the house for being unable to invite guests: no room to cook or sit down.

Emotional effects:

Idealises hd. Feels her life is effectively over. Loss has reactivated grief for her mother (d. 1969) and a miscarriage (1955).

Social situation

Son lives nearby; visits two-three times a week, but

friction with his girlfriend.

Dau visits c. once a month with granddaughter; phone contact in between.

Social contacts through church; visits brother (blind; brain damaged; in residential care) each week; a few widowed friends.

Finances

Church pension + OAP; savings went into house. Poor financial management. Says she never saw an electricity bill until hd died ('and no wonder he used to get so upset about them'). Problems with car.

Client's expressed needs

More money, better housing, better health.

Unlikely to accept counselling help: 'Nothing will bring back' hd. Meanwhile 'will get by somehow'. Clings to her professional status as vicar's wife. Talks to friends and family. Frightened of doctors.

This grim picture had little impact on me. This was just the way my mother was. I had even let Kathy go and stay with her from time to time while she still wanted to. It was only much later that Kathy told me about getting up in the night once when she was about five and going downstairs. Didi was sitting at the kitchen table and poured her a coke – then offered her some whisky to go in it.

I went over and over the story of Deidre's miscarriage, trying to understand what had actually happened, and why my feelings about it were still so acute, even though I had recovered from my own. I had only what she had told me, and Pete's memories. I did know that I slept in a dressing room off my parents' bedroom. There are many things I might have heard – or even seen – that night. Afterwards I had tried so hard to make it all right that I imagined the baby, and used to help it downstairs behind me.

The idea of magical thinking as a developmental phase leapt out of a book I was reading. A child of three experiences herself as the centre of the universe, and therefore attributes events in the outside world to her own desires, without ascribing objective causes to them. So, for example, a child fantasises her baby brother is dead. This may be quite normal, and passes – but if the baby *does* die, the child might believe that it was her desire that killed him. This, I reckoned, had happened to me: I had eaten the beautiful glass butterfly given by my father to my mother and it had etched a deep and ineradicable guilt on my soul.

I struggled to imagine how it might have been, that night.

She has a baby inside her ... everyone is excited ... I think I like the idea of a baby – like a doll only alive. ... I like the idea of protecting it, cuddling it, playing with it. Perhaps in some way I feel that it will be my *baby.*

Mummy looks a bit fatter because the baby's inside her, all safe and cared for inside her tummy. I wonder what it feels like to be safe and cared for inside someone, and what it's like to come out ... Do I want to get closer to Mummy and cuddle her a lot to make sure there is room for me? The baby's all right. It's safe and sound inside where nothing can harm it.

I like getting in bed with Mummy in the morning and having a saucer of her tea – 'cup-of-tea-in-a-saucer'. I can smell the bed now. It is a good, comfort-

ing smell. Is there room in it for all of us and a baby?

Is Mummy worried about the baby? No. She's excited. She's happy.

Then, suddenly, she's gone. She left the baby behind in the bed and he's not safe anymore because he came out too soon ... The bed is full of a dead baby – not so much a baby as a sort of fishy thing – and there is a lot of blood.

Where is everyone? I am sure that Nana is here somewhere, looking after us but I can't see her.

What happened? Why? Who did it?

Did the baby do it? Did I tell it to come out because I wanted to play with it? Or because I didn't want it taking up all the space inside my Mummy?

Did I do it while I wasn't looking? The same way I ate the glass butterflies in the dream?

Suppose no-one killed the baby. Suppose it just died, like Nana. I didn't kill it. My mother didn't kill it. My father didn't kill it. It just died.

Why the hell couldn't someone say so!

Trying to see the story from the perspective of a three year old, I learned to care for and reassure my child self as though she were my own daughter – a technique that would stand me in good stead ten years further on. I sat down with this three year old self and spoke to her, trying to explain that none of it was her fault.

It's not that she doesn't love you. Your Mummy is so unhappy inside herself that she can't see you at the moment. If she could see you it would help her to feel better. She does love you, but she is all wrapped up in something terribly sad that is awful for her, but it is also awful for you because you are shut out of it.

You feel bad because you need her love and can't get it, not because you are bad. I know you are not bad because I know you love her and wanted to love the baby. Your Mummy can't let go of the baby – not because there is something extra special about the baby but because of other things she's never been able to let go of, like her Daddy who died when she was little. But I can let that baby go and I have the right to do that for you because I love you and I can see you, and I have had a baby and lost a baby so I know what has to be done ....

As you got older, you needed to become independent, but you were so aware of this huge hole inside your mother that you learned to disguise yourself. You couldn't fill the hole – whatever you did was wrong ...

As this work went on, I began to understand – and somehow rearrange – the feelings inside me. The changes felt physical. Listening to music, or simply lying on the floor trying to hold myself from falling through it, I could feel movements inside me which seemed to me like the shifting of tectonic plates beneath the earth's crust. 'There are such huge movements', I wrote in my journal, 'that every few hours I have to dip into this molten swirling and draw some up into consciousness.'

During the analysis I also reproduced all the symptoms of the duodenal ulcer I had had when I was fifteen. My GP arranged a scan, but it showed up nothing. I told her about the therapy, and she seemed rather doubtful about whether it was a good thing. The pain inside became concentrated into what I experienced as the sponge like thing I had felt inside me when talking with Mr O. Now it was hardened, smaller - ' a horrible, raw pulsating thing'.

Then one day it was outside me.

Its presence was completely real to me, even while I knew it did not actually exist. I inspected it, without attempting to touch it, and made notes on what I saw:

> *... a floppy, slippery thing, that might make you laugh if you tried to pick it up. But also terrifying. To touch it would cause such pain. Whose pain?*

> *I have felt this thing inside me as a threat which underlies everything I have become, but which, if uncovered, could drown all that in a scream.*

> *It is also Eliot's 'infinitely gentle, infinitely suffering thing' – always there, always patient.*

> *I have protected it – from myself, from other people – unable to bear the thought of its pain if it were touched.*

> *I have feared it because its pain is also my pain: pain that could wipe me out. I have resented it pulsating inside me, raw and painful.*

> *In the last few days I have noticed it is outside me. It is not in my mother, either, but on the floor. It is not only not in her: it is not in me either. I have chucked it out, like a frisbee, and there it is on the floor. I could weep for joy. It is not mine any longer.*

For a week or two, wherever I was, in Jim's office, in church or in my study, I was almost hysterical with joy because that thing – that floppy, red, pulsating, *joke* which had had me fooled for years – was out there, on the floor, a few feet away from me. Day by day it calmed down. It slowly lost its life, while I said goodbye to it as to a long standing companion. Then it was gone.

3

A New Career

THERE WAS NO DOUBT Patricia and I did good work together. But I did fall into my usual trap: the achievement trap.

It was part of the family legend that when I began school at four I did not speak a single word for the whole of the first term. The teachers had no idea I could already read. They called in my parents and suggested I might need special education. My mother thought this was a great joke.

Whatever was said to me, from then on I worked hard and did well. I was the clever one who could pass exams; Pete was the creative one who made them irrelevant. Yet although I enjoyed academic work, relationships mattered more. If there was no one I wanted to please, I was not much interested.

Pete dropped out of university and had a series of jobs on buildings sites, in garages and so on, but he had published two novels. I dipped a toe into social work and then teaching, though I qualified in neither of them, and ended up working in Jim's business. By the time 'the thing' ejected itself from my psyche, this work had become depressing: every time I walked into his office I felt as though a large black hat descended onto my head. It was partly that we had very different ideas about how to run things – and it was his business, not mine. It also meant different things to each of us: for me it was a means to an end – the hope of being able to live without lodgers and have more children – but for him it was an end in itself.

The business operated on an all-or-nothing culture where deadlines could mean staying up all night; by having a baby and going part time I inevitably found myself marginalised. Because I had a child to look after and had to have my computer in one place or the other (this was well before laptops), I worked mostly in our living space upstairs. It soon became clear to me why working at home had not caught on as much as you might expect in the computer age. Working at home there is none of the *camerarderie* of office life. There is only the work – and I had all the jobs nobody else wanted: the admin, the accounts, the marketing. The business was taking over my time, my home and my husband, and I no longer felt part of it.

All my life I had thrived on goals and now I lacked one. After a few months of seeing Patricia, however, I began to work hard at therapy.

I was good at therapy. After a year or two of working together, Patricia encouraged me to go into training myself. I was accepted by CRUSE to train and then volunteer as a bereavement counsellor. From there I went on to train as a therapist; my therapy with Patricia now had the added dimension of being part of my training. I was still experiencing and learning to manage deep feeling, but also with a view to being able to contain other people's.

I devoured the literature – Jung, Freud, Winnicott, Klein and their later derivatives. Each of the theories made sense in their own way – Jung and Carl Rogers most of all.

Case histories could be problematic, however. Reading about other people's experience often made me feel affirmed and understood, but there were times when I simply felt betrayed. I would be reading an account that seemed like what went on in me, making me feel less isolated, and then there would be a sudden distance: 'Of course, in extreme cases ...'; 'When a patient is really disturbed...': phrases that went on to describe something that sounded just like me. Take Anthony Storr, for example:

> The more deeply disturbed the patient ... the more likely it is that the therapist will be exalted to the position of being 'the only person who understands'.

Was that not me with Patricia? I did not just 'view her in a positive light' – an aspect of the therapeutic relationship that Storr regarded as essential: she had become my model, my ideal, someone whose presence or absence felt like the difference between life and death.

Patricia was at the heart of a thriving local network of experienced therapists who wanted to see their tradition continued and who nurtured their protégés well. I was drawn into this circle, finding there mentors and colleagues as well as stimulating discussion, and being part of the group also helped me helped me build my practice. Andrew, another Jungian analyst, agreed to become my supervisor. Initially intimidating, he turned out to be a nurturing, quixotic and deeply interesting man. I had, as it were, two good parents in place, and several 'siblings.' It was a heady time, finding myself welcomed and accepted among these people, several of whom became lasting friends. It was, I thought, how it should have been at Oxford if I had not been in such a withdrawn state when I was a student there.

Still an achiever, I came out of my training with flying colours and was offered the opportunity to do a doctorate, to 'get on the conference circuit', even to help one of the tutors set up an M.A. course in another part of the country. But I was well provided for in my home surroundings, and I wanted to get on with the job. It was also time to end – reluctantly – with Patricia. I was her colleague now.

In five years we had delved as deeply as we could into my relationship with my mother, but any attempts to talk about my father got stuck. I remained deeply attached to him – or rather to the memory of him – but I simply could not access who he was or what our relationship really had been like. It was difficult, too, to disentangle him as a person from the Church, though my current developing church life was helping me to do that. Just after I finished working with Patricia, I had a dream about St George's:

> *I am outside my father's church and start to go in to have a look at it. As I do so, something stirs in the dark of the porch. I am terrified and run away. I hear Pete's voice saying, 'Don't go in there. Why put yourself through that?'*

It would be another seven years before I would understand this dream. Meanwhile, I knew that this was a time to be treasured. Jim was getting older, my mother was coping less and less well in her home, Kathy would leave at some point. Referring to the Egyptian famine in the time of Joseph, I said to Father Richard one day, 'I think of these as my seven fat years. I need to store them up for what is to come.'

Even so, things were not easy at home. I had not realised how much my marriage relied on my having no interests outside the business, and now it rapidly deteriorated. I had hoped that Jim would be freer and happier running his business his own way without me, and that by forging a new and satisfying career path – which did, after all, contribute to the family finances – I would come to have a better and more equal relationship with him. This did not happen. We continued to live – and sleep – together, but our waking lives moved onto parallel tracks. This was sad and difficult for both of us, but I loved having an adolescent daughter whose many friends were regularly in and out of the house, and I loved my working life.

You could say that I was somewhat driven, but the system worked. I built my practice, lectured in psychology, wrote articles, brought up my daughter and made many good friends. Patricia and I had done a pretty good job. I now knew first hand that there was such a thing as healing, and that for some people this was achieved by the talking cure – or rather, I would have said, by a quality of reliable attention combined with honesty and a little insight here and there. The analysis and the training had both been deep and healing experiences.

In spite of all this, I was still capable of waking up shouting in terror after a nightmare:

I am in St George's, near the entrance, trying to help a man (a priest?) with a task. We can't get on with it because there is a mad man in the vestry, and we will probably have to get help. The man/priest has a friend, a psychiatrist called Russell Lockheart who knew the madman and might have to be called.

There are noises coming from the vestry, and the man/priest sends me across the road to phone from a call box in the Tube station. The call boxes are right inside the station, which is deserted and I feel scared and trapped. And then I can't get an answer.

At last Russell Lockheart's wife picks up the phone and we have some agonisingly slow social chat before I can ask if he is at home. She says, 'Yes, he's at home,' and goes to fetch him, but doesn't come back. Meanwhile, I can hear or sense a big man coming into the station in slow, measured steps. I am blind in the light and cannot see him, but I know he is coming for me.

I start screaming down the phone in case Russell Lockheart can hear me.

Russell was the name of a psychiatrist who had been a member of my father's parish. And 'Lockheart' had done an efficient job inside me. Whose side, I was to wonder later, was he on?

Part 3
BACK TO THE FAMILY:
DEATH, ALCOHOL
AND UNCLE JIMMY

*His craving for alcohol was the equivalent on a
low level of the spiritual thirst of our being for
wholeness ... for the union with God.*
C.G. Jung: Letter to Bill Wilson

1

Alcohol Vanquished

SOME MONTHS AFTER I had finished my training and not long
after I stopped seeing Patricia, I had a phone call from Pete.

He, too, was now in therapy with a Jungian, and we
often talked about Jung and about therapy in general. Pete
had at last found a niche with a small Arts co-operative
which enabled him to work mainly at home and find time to
write. His partner, Jeanine, worked in a PR firm in the city
so he had the house pretty much to himself on weekdays.
Since we both had flexible hours we met up now and then
during the week, as well as speaking on the phone. Even so
I had the impression that the Pete I knew was only the tip

of the iceberg: much of his life went on out of sight of any of us.

He still saw Deidre two or three times a week, and seemed to hold a mysterious knowledge of her in which I was not included. One Christmas, worried as always about Deidre's finances, and knowing she liked whisky, I asked Pete if I should get her a case of Scotch for Christmas. He looked at me in a worried way, and said, 'I wouldn't do that if I were you.'

Pete's close relationship with Deidre was just fine by me: it let me off the hook. I phoned her most weeks, and saw her as regularly as I could – mainly on my own. Now that Kathy found her almost as difficult as I did I wanted to shield her, and since Kathy had started growing up Deidre seemed less interested anyway. Did that happen with me, too? I wondered. *No room for a young woman in that house*.

There was no doubt, though, that since Hugh died Pete had found Deidre much more of a struggle. It was as though Hugh had provided a filter that was no longer there, and I knew Pete no longer stayed close because he wanted to so much as because he felt he had to – or perhaps because he found it harder than me to break away.

Pete's phone call came late one evening when I was in my study catching up on some paperwork. It was unusual for him to phone in the evening.

'Are you on your own?' he asked.

'Yes'.

'I've something I need to tell you,' he said, 'but it is strictly confidential between you and me. Don't even tell Jim.'

'OK.'

There was a pause in which I ran through possibilities of terminal cancer, an arrest, a break-up with Jeanine. Much as I loved Pete, I was always relieved that I did not have to live with him. Then Pete spoke. 'I'm a recovering alcoholic,' he said.

In a way it was no surprise. For as long as I could remember I had had a vague dread that he would end up in a gutter like Deidre's father. Pete's drinking had been notorious since his teens. He once broke the nose of a friend who tried to stop him driving home from a party. Another time he was brought home by the police with his face bruised by their truncheons after they picked him up on the main road. He had been throwing cardboard boxes at the passing cars to make them stop so he could tell them about Vietnam. It was after a drinking session with Hugh's curate that he went around the further reaches of the parish in the small hours looking for a 'a nice old couple' that would take him in, and woke up hours later in a dustbin.

Even so, the word 'alcoholic' was something else. I had not realised until now that he needed a quarter of spirits to start the day, or that his teeth and his hands had already been damaged by alcohol.

'I always dreaded Lent,' Pete told me, 'even though I wasn't at church, because I always told myself I would give up alcohol for Lent. By mid-morning on Ash Wednesday I'd be thinking, "I'll give up spirits for Lent", and have a Guinness. By lunchtime it would be "I'll give up being drunk by the time Jeanine gets home" – for Lent.'

As for 'recovering', this had begun with his therapist. One

day when he turned up to his ten a.m. session with a quarter of whisky inside him, she put him straight into her car and drove him to his GP. By some means the GP got him straight away to Alcoholics Anonymous, and from that day he never drank again. Sober, Pete was grateful to his therapist, but, he told me, 'If I had had a gun that morning I would have shot her.'

It was an impressive story. I could not imagine myself doing what she had done.

The 'Anonymous' component to AA was crucial, Pete told me. That was why he did not want me to tell anyone, even Jim.

'What happens,' he said, 'is that if people know you are not drinking they can't resist trying to get you to have just one drink. So if there are family things – Christmas and stuff – you need someone there who knows, but the rest of the people not to know. You're my ally now when I'm not drinking at parties and things and like that. We say "recovering" because an alcoholic is an alcoholic. There is no such thing as "just one drink".'

For the rest of his life Pete went to meetings – daily for the first few years – wherever he was. He always carried the Twelve Steps with him and followed it religiously, and became a sponsor for other recovering alcoholics. I had my church and he had his.

Being Pete, he watched himself doing all this, and entertained me with stories of alcoholic cunning: burying cans of Special Brew in allotments, hiding quarters of spirits in lavatory cisterns. And though his life depended on it he was also amused by the addictive power of the Twelve Steps.

'In America, now,' he told me, 'they even have Twelve

Steps groups to help you recover from the Twelve Steps.'

I thought I had gone into my own story pretty thoroughly, but alcohol was so much a part of family life that I hadn't really thought about it. Always in the background was the shadow of Deidre's father who had 'drunk himself to death' when she was seven. All I knew was that when they were homeless because his business had failed, Nana's sister Flo had temporarily taken in her and the children but refused to have my grandfather in the house. He died on the streets of emphysema. Deidre had been sent to school on the day of the funeral. She had one sepia photograph of him – a handsome man with a moustache, and on the rare occasions when she talked about him, she presented him as a gentle, romantic poet.

I never heard Nana talk about him. Pete remembered her telling a story about our grandfather spending his last bit of money on a bottle of Guinness. They lived then in a basement flat in Mirthyr Terrace, and as he came down the area steps he slipped and dropped the bottle. It smashed on stone at the bottom the steps.

'It was *Murder* Terrace that night', Nana told Pete.

When we were growing up there was never a day when our parents did not drink at lunch time and in the evening. Deidre was always anxious if people could not have what they wanted. She worried when certain people went into hospital, and on at least one occasion smuggled in whisky disguised in a Lucozade bottle. She always packed a half bottle of Scotch in Hugh's suitcase when he went on his annual five days' retreat, but Hugh, we concluded, was not a full blown alcoholic.

'He didn't drink just anything,' said Pete. 'He cared about good wine'.

Deidre was another matter. Pete knew far more about her habits than I did, and now they began to fall into place. The reason she stayed up after everyone else was to do her serious drinking, and she only really cared for whisky. It was one reason, Pete explained, why she so loved the amphetamines, the little yellow pills. They masked any hangover the next morning.

Alcoholism, he explained to me, was an illness, and you could see the gene passing through our family from our grandfather to our mother to him. It had missed me, he reckoned: although I drank regularly, I was not a sitting duck for alcoholism.

Pete's experience fed into my teaching, and my lectures on alcoholism became detailed and thorough. In his correspondence with Bill Wilson, the founder of AA, Jung remarked that it may be no accident that we refer to alcoholic drinks as 'spirits'. I was able to speak with conviction about the relationship between Spirit and spirit, and the vulnerability of certain people to addiction. I could see that liminal, creative quality in Pete, and even in my mother. I suspected my grandfather had it too.

2

Uncle Jimmy

PETE HAD BEEN SOBER for about a year when it became clear that my mother's life was coming apart. Her depression was palpable, like a lead weight that followed her around and sat where she sat.

'When she comes to visit,' said Kathy one day, 'it feels as though she brings a black hole with her and tries to suck everyone into it.' Like me, Kathy felt helpless. In the work with Mr O., I had begun to understand that the place where my mother would be happy did not exist.

As I had noted in my 'social work report' five years before, Deidre had had to leave her home within a few months of Hugh dying. The five bedroom vicarage was heavily silted up, and Pete and I tried to help her sort her belongings, a task of Herculean proportions. Every black sack we filled for the charity shop or the garbage she opened up again, poured the contents on the floor and decided to keep ninety per cent of it: broken toys, torn comics, battered crucifixes, old clothes, pieces of string .....

Even she had to agree to part with some furniture, but everything else was crammed into her two-up, one-down terrace, along with a summerhouse and shed which were both stuffed from floor to ceiling. Somehow the substantial legacies left by Hugh's parents in the 1960s had trickled away. I, a lecturer on co-dependency, was paying her mortgage.

I forced myself to visit Deidre once a month. The doorbell was usually out of order, so I would knock on the door, or shout through the letterbox. Each time it seemed to take longer for her to respond, and I stood on the doorstep torn between hope and dread: dread of her opening the door; hope – and dread – that she would not. Finally there would be a scrabbling sound on the far side of the door as she took off the chain and undid the mortice lock, swearing a bit as her fingers grappled with the keys. Then she was there, bedraggled, cross, anxious, her face stretched in an attempt at a smile. It was years since we had hugged or touched each other.

Every conceivable surface in the house, including the floor and the stairs, was covered with junk. Deidre refused ever to open the heavy green velvet curtains over the windows on the street side of the house, so dim light bulbs burned all day. There were weird echoes of the vicarage in the row of Home Pride Flour men still peeking out from among grimy papers and cups on a shelf in the kitchen, and the photos of religious figures and politicians she had stuck on the bathroom wall with a note inviting people to add their own captions. Pete had even written a few.

At some point during each visit, I would try to do the washing up that was heaped up in the kitchen sink. After the first few layers you came to black slime, and increasingly I simply gave up, feeling guilty for leaving it. JESUS LOVES YOU screamed a sticker on the fridge door.

And I couldn't even do a bit of washing up for my mother. She was also running out of storage space for the empty bottles. They already filled the larder but she would not let me put them out with the rubbish. 'If I put them out for the dustmen,' she said, 'they might find them and accuse me of being an alcoholic.' ('That *would* be a pity, wouldn't it' remarked Pete when I told him.)

I could not see how anyone could prepare or eat food there, so I used to take Deidre out for dinner at a local motel. She had many falls and bruises, and one time when I arrived to take her out, she had a black eye.

'What happened to your eye?' asked the waitress at the motel.

'I fell on the stairs,' my mother replied.

The waitress tossed her head and laughed.

'Nonsense! You've got a new boyfriend.'

I was an experienced driver and used to finding my way around, but every time I came away from Deidre's house, desperate to get home to Jim and Kathy, to civilisation as I knew it, I would get lost. It took anything up to half an hour to find my way out of the suburban streets and head for the motorway. Only then did I put on Bob Dylan at full blast to power me home. *You say you're lookin' for someone Never weak but always strong … But it ain't me, babe, No, no, no, … It ain't me you're lookin' for, babe…. I didn't mean to make you so sad … Sooner or later one of us must know…*

My getting lost was particularly strange since Deidre had not moved far from the vicarage, and her house was in familiar territory. Pete explained to me she needed to stay with the same GP practice where they knew about the amphetamines and would go on prescribing them. As the vicar's widow, however, it was not considered appropriate for her to go on going to my father's most recent parish. Instead she went back to St George's, the first parish Pete and I remembered.

We were both upset about this, for reasons that amounted to no more than a vague sense of dread. We had both done our best to forget that church and its parishioners, and now they began to surface from the depths. Pete was inclined to the picaresque when he talked about it. I, as my mother had noted at Hugh's funeral, tended to clam up.

Pete was the first to realise what was happening and he immediately warned me. 'It is unbelievable. She's going to St George's on Sundays now. They are all still there. All those corpses and vampires of our childhood are suddenly starting to crawl out of their coffins. Anyone else would have been long dead, but not them. They are all still there.'

For us these people had lived an unimaginably long time ago. It was inconceivable that they should still be alive, but they were, of course, around the same age as Deidre — in their early seventies. While for us they had ceased to exist, they had simply gone on living in the same area and attending church. Their names started to surface in our mother's conversation, not as memories but as realities. She spoke as though we would be pleased to have news of them, but they stirred up feelings which neither of us wanted. It never occurred to us that our reactions were odd. This was simply the way we felt, and had always felt as long as we could remember.

'Can you believe,' Pete rang to say, 'She's been to tea with Mrs Turner?'

'Mrs Turner? Didn't she do the flowers? Surely she

must be dead by now?'

'Afraid not. Yes, she was always running around with dead dahlias, looking for some stinking heap of compost where she could leave their slimy remains.' There was a reflective pause. 'What I remember about Mrs Turner, is her sneaking up on me when I was playing behind the church one day. She half scared the life out of me. I had an awful sense of shame as if she had caught me out in some ghastly act, and I am sure that I was not committing one – not that time, anyway. Thank Christ no-one calls me 'Peter' anymore.'

As for the children of these people, they had of course become vicars or bankers or doctors, or charming housewives who kept nice houses and loved their mothers.

'I remember Sally,' said Pete, after Deidre referred wistfully to one of these paragons, 'She used to tie me to the apple tree and whip me with saplings. I quite liked it.'

I, too, could picture that apple tree, and remembered Pete tying *me* to it, and using me as target practice for his home-made bow and arrow.

Pete had many more memories than I did. 'There were those two enormously fat jelly-like old ladies with the underground flat. Do you remember who they were?' he asked.

'Not a clue.'

'The flat smelt of cats. *She'* (Pete usually referred to Deidre as 'She' or 'Her'; she disliked her own name and refused to use it, so neither of us were quite sure what to call her since we had stopped saying 'Mummy') '*She* didn't like going there. I was gripped by tremendous anxiety from the briefing on the way there – what trouble I'd be in if I didn't behave nicely and "showed my mother up" – do you remember that whole thing about "showing her up"?'

'Tell me some more' I said, drawn into the narrative, but with my own memory a blank.

'I remember snatching off my cap as one of the old Jellies opened the door and having a huge sense of relief. By remembering to remove the school cap, I'd done something right!'

I could see Pete in his dark green school cap with its red and black trim. The first time he went to see his therapist, he told me, her children's blazers and caps were hanging in the hall. They went to the same school we had gone to, and the sight of their uniforms gave him a panic attack.

'Some therapy that was,' he remarked. 'But the old ladies – the Jellies. There was a huge gloomy hallway and as we approached the inner sanctum the stink of cats increased. They lived with a bunch of malodorous felines which used to perch on the back of the sofa and hiss as we went in. What I mainly remember is trying desperately hard to be polite, non-existent and good. If I succeeded I didn't get a terrible telling off on the way home. That was one of *Her* favourite tricks. No word of correction if you were being naughty while you were out: just this terrible unexpected *Stuka* attack on the way home.'

'Yeah,' I said, 'That rings a bell. She'd smile at you while you were somewhere, and you would think it was going all right. And then suddenly it hadn't.'

The other end of the phone I could feel Pete shudder. 'Christ, the anxiety and terror of all that.'

Nevertheless, in her own way our mother had kept going after Hugh died. Now, however, she was showing signs of dementia, and what scared us more than anything was that she was still driving. She went everywhere by car because she had always been terrified of public transport – another thing we simply took for granted – but we had seen her in action and knew she was a danger on the road. There were news stories of old ladies hitting the wrong pedal and driving into crowded shopping streets, children ... She could end up as one of them and how would we live with ourselves if we had sat by and done nothing?

Deidre particularly needed the car to visit our Uncle Jimmy. Born in 1917, Uncle Jimmy was delivered with forceps which grasped his head in the wrong place: as a result he was brain damaged, blind and epileptic.

Nana went on to have two more children, our Uncle Paddy and Deidre. After her husband died, Nana somehow scraped together a home and a living for them all. She would never talk about it when I asked because she was 'ashamed' of the jobs she had done in kitchens and factories. I could never understand how she could be ashamed of working her fingers to the bone to support her family. Meanwhile, the children had to become what my mother called 'latch key kids' – something she was determined should never happen to us – and she never went out to work.

Deidre and Paddy had equal and opposite reactions to Jimmy. Paddy was nothing but angry, and he taunted Jimmy mercilessly, goading him into the rages that eventually meant Nana could no longer keep him at home. Deidre adored Jimmy and was eaten up with guilt that he could not have a normal life; she longed for a miracle that would restore his sight. On one occasion when the three children went together to the local park, Paddy helped Jimmy climb a tree. He then walked away into the dusk, leaving Deidre at the bottom of the tree and Jimmy stranded on a branch. It was Deidre who managed to coax Jimmy down and lead him home. And it was Deidre who told me these things. Nana never spoke about any of it.

As he grew into adolescence Jimmy became more and more difficult to manage. Deidre went along with him and Nana on visits to doctors who said things like, 'If I had had him when he was a small child... ' or 'If they had known then what they know now ...' But the message was always the same: too late, too late, too late.

Eventually Jimmy's fits and his rages of frustration – fuelled by Paddy – became more than Nana and Deidre could handle, and at seventeen he went to live in a residential hospital some distance out of London. As long as I could remember we all visited every Wednesday. Deidre and Hugh kept it up after Nana died and we left home, and now Deidre did it on her own. Pete went now and then to see him, and I very occasionally. I would have sent regular postcards, but Deidre thought that was a bad idea: it would be so disappointing for him if I forgot or stopped doing it.

When we were children the hospital stank of urine, everyone slept in dormitories and the regime was strict. On the terrace outside the ward on a summer day there would be a line of wheelchairs. We tried not to look at the large pram in which lay curled up a middle aged man the size of a child. Uncle Jimmy was one of the lucky ones. He was able to walk around and do simple work in the workshops.

Uncle Jimmy himself was a gentle giant. For some reason he had never learned to use a white stick, so if he walked anywhere he did so holding on to someone's arm or hand. He was a big man and it was very slow. The more active patients would follow us around the grounds and wheedle for change to spend in the canteen. At some point the hospital started paying a small wage for the work Uncle Jimmy did, and then there was constant anxiety about this being stolen by patients who could see.

Three times a year Uncle Jimmy would come 'home' for two or three days, and while he was staying with us Deidre always wanted him to have some sherry or lager. He had pills for epilepsy and Nana and my father worried that you were not supposed to have alcohol with them. We never really knew whether Deidre had given him the pills or not – and Pete and I would hold our breath while she gave Uncle Jimmy his glass of sherry. We had been told what to do if he had a fit, but I did not want to see him flailing about and foaming at the mouth. He was also on tranquilisers and when there was doubt about which pills he had actually taken there were dark remarks about what might happen without them.

Meanwhile, he had to be kept occupied. Deidre got out the record player and played his 78 rpm records which were kept in a special cupboard: *Davey Crockett, King of the Wild Frontier.., Felix Kept on Walking* … Uncle Jimmy would rock back and forth and make singing sounds, while Deidre kept up a running commentary on how musical he would have been if only…. She banned any romantic songs because he had never had a love life. He liked to help with polishing, and I dreaded the moment when he would polish the piano. Sooner or later he would run the cloth noisily up and down the keys – and Deidre would remark on his long fingers and what a pianist he could have been.

We usually took him out somewhere – a local park or

garden – but we were not allowed to comment on anything we saw. If we did there would be a gentle but devastating reproach. 'Yes the flowers are pretty but Uncle Jimmy can't see them' – *if only, if only, if only*. The second half of the visit was spent in the shadow of his return to the hospital and a frenzy of anxiety about leaving as late as possible but not so late he would get into trouble. Much depended on who would be on duty that evening. Mr Willis was lenient, but Mr Thompson would – we never knew what Mr Thompson would do if we were late, but it would undoubtedly be unpleasant. Deidre never let Uncle Jimmy disappear from our minds. Even at the dentist we were told to 'Offer up the pain for Uncle Jimmy'.

As for Uncle Paddy, he resolutely refused to go anywhere near the hospital though he would sometimes drop in when Uncle Jimmy was 'home' with us, and make remarks about cripples which sent Deidre muttering into the scullery. He became a police inspector, and was so renowned for racism and sadism that the local people held a street party when he retired – not in his honour.

In time the hospital where Uncle Jimmy lived improved dramatically. The residents began to be treated as people rather than patients, and the buildings became homely and friendly, with more privacy. There were art and music workshops as well as the occupational therapy work. In his fifties Uncle Jimmy was confirmed and started to go to communion, something that would previously have been unthinkable for someone with his level of learning difficulty. He was delighted, and looked forward to it every week. On one occasion when he fell in the bath he saw it as being accepted into suffering because of his love. 'It's because I love Jesus so much,' he said.

I passionately believed that in society as it now was, it did not have to be so bad to be Uncle Jimmy. If he could be accepted as he was, the fact that he was loved and cared for in the hospital and regularly visited by his family could be experienced as some sort of triumph of good over the undoubted evil of his injury.

Not if Deidre had anything to do with it. Uncle-Jimmy-filtered-by-Deidre remained unbearable. After Hugh died, she became consumed with guilt that she did not have him to live with her permanently. She still had him 'home' for short holidays and our aunt Cordelia, Hugh's sister, went too to make it possible. She told me that she had promised this to Hugh before he died. We avoided talking too much about what these stays were like. I only knew that I could not have done it, though both Pete and I both made a point of inviting them all to our houses during the visits, to give Cordelia a breath of outside air.

As for the Wednesday visits, there was no public transport from where Deidre lived to the hospital even if she would have used it, and no way Deidre was going to stop driving. Pete tried giving up an afternoon a week to take her. He could not get away on Wednesdays, but he could manage Tuesdays. It was only after a few weeks he discovered that she still went on Wednesdays as well.

'She said she could not bear to think of him without a Wednesday visit after all these years. Fucking hell. We had been there on fucking Tuesday.'

Jeanine, Pete's partner, was also furious. She, after all, had to cope with Pete's depression after the weekly ordeal. 'Jeanine actually went round there and shouted at her. She called her a stupid old woman' Pete told me.

I could hardly take this in. 'What happened?'

'Well, nothing.' She just told her to get out and slammed the door behind her.

'I can't believe it.' Pete knew what I meant. Jeanine had called Deidre a stupid old woman and the sky had not turned black, the world had not gone up in flames. On reflection I realised that Deidre would know exactly how to deal with it. It was just one more piece of evidence that it was 'that Jeanine' who was ruining her relationship with Pete.

I was free on Wednesdays and said I would try doing a visit once a month. I drove to London, picked up Deidre and drove on to the hospital, where they were welcoming and pleased to see us. It was hardly like a hospital these days, with day rooms and bright colours. We took Uncle Jimmy out for tea and a slow, ambling walk in the park in a nearby town. He leaned heavily on Deidre who could barely walk herself, so I took his arm. *It's not really so bad*, I told myself once they were both back in the car and we were on the way back to the hospital. *I can do this.* We were almost there when Deidre asked me stop in a layby. It was getting dark and it had begun to rain, and cars – cars full of normal people going about a normal day – swished past us.

Uncle Jimmy was sitting beside me and she was in the back, where it turned out she had a large bag full of food and drink. It was a scene I had witnessed all my life, a kind of reverse image of taking candy from a baby. Anything you offered Jimmy he would accept. I sat frozen behind the steering wheel as Deidre set about it. 'Jimmy, would you like a ham sandwich?'

'Yes please, Deidre.'

'Jimmy, would you like a drink of beer?'

'Yes please, Deidre.'

'Would you like a bit more cake?'

With each thing Deidre passed through from the back of the car a further layer of stickiness attached itself to Uncle Jimmy's fingers, his mouth and his surroundings. From time to time Deidre reached forward and wiped around his mouth with a damp rag she had brought in a plastic bag.

At last it came to an end. Then, as we arrived at the hospital gates Uncle Jimmy was sick all over the inside of my car. I did not go again.

Pete and I did manage, however, to get Uncle Jimmy reclassified as fit for ordinary 'Part III' – old people's home – accommodation, and he was moved to a home around the corner from where Deidre was living. At eighty, for the first time in his life, he had a room of his own.

3

Alcohol Triumphant

Boy, you're going to carry that weight, carry that weight a long time .....

The Beatles

ONE DAY I ARRIVED at Deidre's house to find that the living room looked as though a wild animal had been let loose in it. A large carriage clock lay smashed on the floor surrounded by other debris. Deidre had no idea how it had happened. There was no sign of any break in. In the end we had to conclude that only she could have done it. Pete found this less strange than I did.

In general I was finding visits a bit easier, since Deidre was not up to talking much. Our best moments were when we sat together in silence.

Though she could get lost for four hours on a trip to the corner shop, Deidre was expert at keeping any kind of helper out of her home – even the GP. Pete and I were the only people she allowed in, apart from a very few people from Hugh's parishes.

One of these was Fred, who for several years had had a room in the vicarage and looked after the garden in return for rent. He was someone else I had not thought about for a long time. He came to live in our house after a divorce, and was always in the kitchen chatting with my mother and commenting on what I ate. Deidre felt sorry for him because his wife hated him so much. 'Do you know,' she said to me, 'she hoovers the whole room but leaves the area around his chair?' She seemed delighted to be able to offer asylum from such a terrible woman.

The summer after Nana died, I was in the outhouse behind the kitchen when Fred came in. He pushed me up against the wall and started putting his hand down inside my trousers. I was at a loss as to what to do. Apart from anything else he was a big man. 'My mother will be home soon,' I said hopefully – and at that moment the front door opened and he disappeared.

Later that day I told my parents, and waited for Fred to be asked to leave. Nothing happened. By this time my parents knew that Pete had slept with his girlfriend – a revelation which had caused Hugh to try and send him away to Borneo as a missionary. Now Hugh had got sufficiently used to the idea to take advantage of it and sent Pete, as a man of the world, to talk to Fred. Still nothing happened, and nothing more was said. I made sure I was never alone in the house with him, and by Christmas I was away with Corinna. Now Fred was one of the few people my mother allowed into her house, and she would tell me about his visits as though he was my favourite uncle.

I wrote to Deidre's GP expressing my concerns and requesting that he try and visit her at home. He replied that he could not discuss her case with me because of patient confidentiality. 'Hmmph', said Pete when I told him. 'Patient confidentiality! More like doctor confidentiality. He knows very well that that practice has been prescribing her speed for decades. It's not altogether his fault – they were legal when they started. By the time he came on the scene they had realised the damage they caused and made them illegal, but it was too late to get some people off them.'

Up and down the country, we knew, there were still hundreds of housewives kept going on prescribed speed or tranquilisers, because it was easier than trying to get them off them. One or two of them were my clients.

Pete's worst experience – apart from alcohol – had been with Valium. Once he managed to get off it he never touched it again however bad he felt.

He told me that Deidre's problem now was that amphetamine had simply become unavailable. The doctor had tried prescribing various substitutes, but none of them met her craving. She was fond of Thyroxin, which she was on anyway for an underactive thyroid, and popped one of these whenever she felt tired, which was often. There seemed to be no check at the surgery on how often she needed a repeat prescription. But it was amphetamine, Pete explained, that had masked the alcohol for all these years. It was her 'drug of choice'. Without it, alcohol was her only hope. For months he tried desperately to get her into AA, but she was not interested. Why do something that took away the one thing she really cared about?

In some ways it was a relief the day we found Deidre on the floor. Rather, Pete found her. I was at an early morning weekday service when it suddenly became clear to me I must ring her. I slipped out of church, found a phone box and dialled her number. Pete answered, and told me had just let himself into the house – unlike me he had a key – and found her lying there. While he sent for an ambulance,

I drove to London. The ambulance men were already there, and had clearly done this many times before. This was just as well because by now she was conscious and protesting. I stood by the front door as they carried her out and felt that the way she looked at me might have been the way Christ looked at Peter when the cock crew. I went in the ambulance with her, while Pete followed in his car.

You are not betraying her, I told myself. At last she'll be in the system. She'll get some help.

In A & E, Deidre was put in a curtained cubicle and we went outside so Pete could smoke – I had given up fifteen years earlier but I had one too – and we phoned Jim and Jeanine to let them know what had happened. Then we went back in and waited. After a while we saw a nurse outside Deidre's cubicle signalling to his colleagues. What he did was to mime drinking from a bottle.

'Shit' we said to each other. Strange as it may seem, Pete being himself a recovering alcoholic and me a mental health professional, it was only then that it really sank in that our mother was an alcoholic.

For the next few days we were both monstrously, selfishly angry. How could she give in to depression after the miscarriage when she had us? How could she have chosen alcohol when she had us? Silly questions, of course, but they seemed real at the time, and were part of taking on our new identity as children of an alcoholic mother.

They kept her in hospital and arranged an appointment at the alcohol dependency unit on the far side of the hospital grounds. Pete and I met and went with her, desperate to hear what they would say. We had to wait a bit longer, however, because a strange thing happened on the way across the hospital grounds. We were all transported in an electric vehicle – a kind of milk float – and Deidre, much better for a few days in hospital, was complaining bitterly about having to go for this appointment. The journey seemed to be taking an impossibly long time. Then, suddenly, the hospital driver stopped, put his head in his hands, and said, 'I don't know where I'm going.'

Pete glanced at our mother and raised his eyebrows to me. 'Psychic contagion', he whispered. The appointment was postponed, and eventually took place without us.

Eventually a doctor told us, yes Deidre needed detox, yes there was already some brain damage, yes she had early Korsakoff's syndrome, and no she should not drive and he was writing to the DVLC about this. He did not yet know what long term plans could be made. Were there funds for private care? If not, a psychiatric ward might be the thing – psychogeriatric, rather, given her age.

'Serve her damn well right,' said Pete afterwards. He, too, had a great longing to take her somewhere and leave her there. I just hoped she would be too out of it to notice where she was, though I rather doubted it.

Detox is a strange thing. After demonstrating all the text book symptoms of Korsakoff's syndrome Deidre became well enough to convince the hospital she was a sweet old lady who ate salmon sandwiches for her tea and just occasionally had the odd glass of sherry. Day by ghastly day the news came in, delivered down the phone by the nurses in bright and encouraging tones. She was walking well. She had made a cup of tea in the ward kitchen. She could do stairs. She was able to sign cheques to pay her bills. Soon we would have to have a discharge meeting.

These phone calls fell through my gut like stones. Helpless, our mother would get looked after. Recovered, she would be sent home and the whole cycle would start again. Gradually it dawned on me that this was only the beginning.

It was only when the hospital staff started making plans for discharge that they began to realise what they were up against. Sweet old ladies who ate salmon sandwiches were also expected to welcome daily carers to help them dress, meals on wheels to keep them well nourished, chiropodists, GP's, district nurses, even a community nurse to discuss the drinking. She would have none of it.

By the time we got to the final meeting, everyone was there: the head of the hospital social services and her long suffering assistant who was in charge of the case, three consultants (medical, alcohol dependency, geriatric), the ward sister, physio, occupational therapist, community nurse, a senior social worker from the Borough … . These combined forces were no match for our mother. She sat there, somehow compacted, leaning on a walking stick, and wiped the floor with them through a simple refusal to cooperate. Meanwhile, Pete and I had done our homework on co-dependency, and had made a pact that if she was not prepared to accept help from outside neither would we offer any. We said so – or rather I did.

Our mother responded as though we had presented her with the solution to a long term problem. 'So if I don't have any more to do with you two,' she said, 'I don't have to have any of these other people either?'

Pete walked out then, and he never spoke to her again. It was at that moment that he realised that Deidre and his new found and fragile sobriety were incompatible. He simply could not afford to spend any time with her if he was to remain sober. Apart from anything else he would be drawn into supplying her with alcohol and that was against his AA code of behaviour. I did not resent his decision. It was literally a matter of life and death for him, and I was beginning to realise how much he had carried throughout my years of relative freedom. So I picked up where he left off. Short of actually communicating with her, he did everything he could to support me.

I needed whatever support was going, because when my mother went home and began to ring me up several times a day, it was agony to stick to what we had said at the meeting: only if she would accept some outside help would I go and visit.

Besides Pete, my other great support was Father Richard. He suggested I changed my phone number, but I could not quite bring myself to do that, and although I kept to not visiting, I spoke to her regularly on the phone. Then the 'corpses and vampires' from St George's started ringing up. How could I neglect my poor mother like this? Didn't I realise she was ill? What sort of daughter was I? In the end, I began to tell them it was hopeless because of the alcohol. It didn't get me very far.

'She doesn't even use alcohol' said the first person I tried it with and I put the phone down. That word 'use' had struck me as interesting.

Although Deidre had been banned from driving, and a policeman had been round and taken her licence (a scene even more unimaginable than Jeanine telling her she was a stupid old woman), she continued to use her car. Haunted by visions of children crippled under her wheels, I phoned the police and explained what was going on. Finally I got someone who appeared to know something about it. 'The trouble is,' he said, 'until she actually has an accident, there is nothing we can do. And even then, if she gets up before a sympathetic magistrate, an old lady like that – she'll probably get away with a warning.'

It took about two months to get back to where we had started with the first admission to hospital. Deidre and I found ourselves back in A and E, and again she was admitted. This time Pete and I managed to get the car removed before she came home. He still had a key to her house, but the car keys were not there. There were plenty of coat hangers, though, and Pete knew just how to lever open the window and unlock it with one of those.

'How do you know all this?' I asked.

'It's better you don't know,' he replied tersely.

One of the neighbours walked past on her way home.

'Fixing up your Mum's car are you?' she asked cheerfully. 'She does make us laugh with that car.'

It was a relief when we finished: I could not help thinking that it would not have been good for my career to be arrested for car breaking. Pete made some mysterious arrangements for its disposal.

When Deidre came out of hospital I expected lamentations and rage, but she never said a word, though she must have known it was us. In any case there were plenty of local minicab drivers only too willing to be paid over the odds for a trip to the off-licence, and at this point she could once more walk as far as the corner shop.

These days too, of course, dial-a-bottle made alcohol available at any time of day or night. Pete had complained about this to me many a time. 'In the old days,' he said, 'at least you knew you were safe from closing time till about ten in the morning, but now they keep dropping these bloody leaflets through your door offering to bring alcohol to you at two a.m. – just when you are really longing for it.'

Several more hospital admissions followed, each with the same result: detox, a partial recovery, refusal of any help, a return home and collapse. The intervals got shorter. Then at last she agreed to have some carers visiting her. Within two days they were on the phone saying they could not get access to the house.

I struggled to keep my work on an even keel, kept going by the thought that I was damned if Deidre was going to wreck it for me. Even so, I was full of guilt that I did not invite her to live with us, though as I told myself, there was no reason to ruin Jim and Kathy's lives as well. Also there was no way I could carry on working if we took her in.

'There's your answer then,' said Father Richard when I talked to him about it. I hoped he was right, though I still suspected I was being selfish. Even I could see, however, that I had no right to inflict her on my family more than I was already doing through the constant crises.

One Sunday when I was visiting my mother in hospital, Uncle Jimmy – now living in the local old people's home – was admitted to the same hospital with a major stroke. I took her down to A and E in a wheelchair and we sat there while they wondered what to do with him. It took some time to get them both settled, and it was after midnight before I got away. I stayed the rest of the night with Pete, and drove back through the dawn to do a day's work. A few days later a doctor phoned to ask me whether they should go through some kind of procedure which involved putting tubes into my uncle's digestive system. He was clearly relieved when I said I did not think it sounded a good idea. After that, Jimmy was clearly dying and one day I asked one of the nurses how long he would last.

'That is in God's hands,' she told me. A few years before I would have wanted to hit her, but to my surprise what she said was deeply comforting. She had said it as though she really meant it. Uncle Jimmy died the next day and was buried next to Hugh and Nana. I managed to get Deidre to the funeral in a wheelchair, and thankfully it all happened quietly without any of Hugh's ex-parishioners. My parents had always kept very quiet about Jimmy where the parish was concerned.

Each time Deidre came home she was a bit more frail and demented, and I wondered how long it would be before anyone said she was not safe to go home. I asked a consultant about it, and tried to explain what the home situation was like. After a few minutes he said, 'I do not believe your mother is a danger to herself. The longer we talk the more convinced I am that it is you who are a danger to her.'

The alcohol dependency man was more sympathetic, but his hands were tied. 'You know and I know,' he said, 'exactly what will happen as soon as she goes home. But as far as the medical profession is concerned, alcohol dependency is not an illness. It is a choice. They are only concerned with her state at the time of discharge. What she chooses to do after that is her choice. I wish I could help, but I can't. Your mother is not certifiable, and until she is we have to fit in with her wishes.'

Pete and I were up against a culture which thought about alcoholism in a completely different way from us. We, like AA, saw it as an illness. If, as the medical profession maintained, it was a choice and not an illness, they were powerless to do anything except repeatedly dry Deidre out and send her back home.

When she was sober she scored well on English and arithmetic tests though they said 'Judgement and insight' were 'impaired'. We puzzled over what this meant, and whether it really represented any change from how she had always been. 'But she was always supposed to be really clever, wasn't she?' I asked Pete. He had met me outside the hospital and we were walking in the local park. 'Hugh was always saying things like "Ah, what insight! That rapier brain!" when she said anything. I always thought she must be clever.'

Pete smiled grimly. 'Yeah, but you know what he was like. It is possible he thought she was stupid and was just sending her up.' This was a shocking but suddenly very plausible thought.

Codependency was to have one more great triumph. It was getting close to the point where even the hospital would have to accept that Deidre needed long term care, when she was kidnapped by another vicar's widow, a school friend called Scilla who thought we were neglecting her. I arrived at Deidre's house one day expecting to call an ambulance, and found Scilla and her sister packing Deidre's things while she sat slumped in a chair. I had no choice but to withdraw and they took her to their home in Dorset. Not long after, I received a phone call from Scilla's daughter, a doctor, who was no more happy about Deidre's state of health than I was, and could see her being a burden on her own mother. '*My* mother drinks,' she sniffed, 'but *she* looks after herself.'

After a few days with them Deidre had a major internal haemorrhage and was rushed into their local hospital. Now I had nearly a three hour journey each way in order to visit her. This time her recovery was much more limited, and everyone was at last agreed that she could not go home. So there she was, stranded in hospital miles from home with no-one prepared to take an interest: since she had steadfastly refused to let social services anywhere near her home, she was not 'known' to the social services where she lived; and she was not the responsibility of the social services in Dorset where she was in hospital. Finally, I managed to get her into a nursing home run by the Church of England for clergy and their widows. It was again a good two hour drive from where I lived, but she had her own room and was beautifully looked after. They even gave her a sherry on Christmas Day, and they were very kind to me.

At last I began to relax – though not for long. Deidre could no longer remember how to dial my number but she got fitter residents to phone me: now I had a series of retired vicars and vicars' widows ringing up to say how lonely my mother was. It was just one more form of torture.

Every time I visited she would ask me if Uncle Jimmy was all right, and I would remind her that he had died, and she would think that this was perhaps just as well. I would remind her about the home that he had been moved to, and that he had had a room of his own there. It was like a child's bedtime story that comforted her, that Jimmy had

had a room of his own at last. In summer I took her out in a wheelchair, trying to make sure we did not go anywhere near a place that sold alcohol. She could sniff it out anywhere, and usually did. I would refuse to let her get at any and felt dreadful, knowing I would need a large gin when I got back home.

Home was also where Deidre wanted to be. 'But you can't walk' I said, after I'd wheeled her out one afternoon. 'I'm not so bad,' she said. 'I didn't fall over once while we were out.'

In any case we had had to sell the house to pay the nursing home fees. Emptying it required several skips and then finally house clearers. Of all the thousands of objects, Pete and I kept nothing. Everything to do with her was pain, and neither of us wanted it.

Having once broken the tie that bound him so closely to our mother Pete continued adamant about not seeing her. One night when I was summoned by the nursing home because they thought Deidre was dying, he drove eighty miles to meet me there. 'I'm glad you've come,' I said, and after he – and I – had had a cigarette and nothing further seemed to be happening, I suggested we went in.

'I'm not coming in!' he replied, as though I had said something crazy.

'Then why did you come?'

'I came to support you,' he told me, 'but there's no way I am going in there. The only way I want to see that woman is laid out on a slab.'

Deidre did not die that night. It was one of several false alarms, and two weeks later Pete sent her a Mother's Day card.

From then on as my mother deteriorated I listened again and again to Bach's *Actus Tragicus*: *Gottes Zeit ist die allerbeste Zeit* (God's time is best). It seemed to me unbelievably tender, and each movement ended on an upward lift, a promise of the future. *Ja, komm, Herr Jesu, komm! ... Heute wirst du mit mir im Paradies sein ....* (Come Lord Jesus ... 'Today you will be with me in Paradise.') That cantata was my prayer.

On 3 May 1998, I had a call which clearly was a final one. Kathy came with me to the nursing home, where we found my mother lying in a bed with cot sides, one remaining front tooth dangling out of her mouth, unconscious but muttering anxiously. Kathy was devastated. 'I did not know people could reach such a state of degradation,' she told me.

I encouraged her to say her goodbyes, and phoned for Jim to come and collect her. His arrival was a deep disappointment for the nurses, who hoped he might be my mother's long lost son.

After Kathy and Jim left, the chaplain arrived for a final blessing. He ended with the prayer, 'Go forth O Christian soul ...' in a solemn voice. I was holding my mother's hand and felt her clench mine in terror as his voice deepened to begin that prayer.

As the evening went by and the day nurses went off shift, they each came in to say a final goodbye to Deidre. Then finally we were alone, and as it got dark she became quieter. All day she had been 'chain-stoking': her breathing would stop for a while and then start up again with a kind of rattle. I wondered if this was what she had meant when she said we should listen for the death rattle in Nana's breathing all those years before.

Around ten o'clock, I slipped out to the Little Chef up the road for something to eat, then came back and sat with her in her room, listening to the gentle sounds of the night shift. Across the corridor, a nurse took a cup of tea to a restless patient and stopped to chat with her. It seemed wonderfully comforting. *I hope I have someone like that to look after me when I am old*, I thought. I tried reading St John's Gospel while I sat there but could not concentrate, and the text seemed quite crazy, not poetic at all.

Gradually everything became still. I did not feel alone with my mother. I had a sense of a door open onto a place full of light and love, and that waiting for her and ready to welcome her were my father, somehow restored, and Nana. Decades of misery seemed to fall away from her as I sat there and held her hand through the cot sides. *I always knew I could get close to you*, I thought. *All it took was for you to be unconscious.* As the sky started to lighten and there were the first twitterings of the dawn chorus, I dozed off, still holding her hand. When I woke up she was dead.

Pete and I never talked about that night. In the months that followed I felt very alone and missed the talks we had had after our father died, the joint journeys of exploration into our grief and our shared longing to know who our parents were.

Pete did come to the funeral. He was proud of me because I stood by the coffin and spoke about my mother. Teaching psychology students had taught me how to hold an audience. I pulled no punches about what the illness of alcoholism had done to her life, but I found I was speaking with love. I commented that our mother was being buried in the one place she would wish to be, with her husband, and near her mother and her brother.

Because of the reference to alcohol I got the odd piece of hate mail afterwards from parishioners, but I was glad I had done it, because the vicar's sermon made me sick. He presented her as a wise old woman who had occasionally visited the parish after her husband's death, and guided it with the benefit of her wisdom. He seemed to have forgotten what those visits were like, such as the time she fell over (drunk) in the path of a visiting bishop, split her head open and refused to go home; by the end of the service, I was told, she had bled her way through a whole toilet roll.

At the wake I had organised in the parish hall, Pete charmed the corpses and vampires (the ones that were not cutting us dead) with the suave skill of a vicar's son. 'You can take the boy out of the Bible belt', he told me afterwards, 'but you can't take the Bible belt out of the boy.' He was inclined to drop things, though, and when I gave him a tub of taramasalata to open, he somehow managed to spray it all over the walls.

I registered the death, cleared her room, proved the will. To my surprise the relief that all that suffering was over was flooded with grief. Whatever Deidre was like, she was my mother and my mother had died. In those last few hours I had found a connection that I had missed all my life, and though I knew very well that it would not have been possible if Deidre had gone on living, it hurt to find it only to lose it again. Driving to the nursing home for the last time, I could not stop crying, and pulled over by a phone box to ring a friend from church. She sympathised and I began to feel calmer. Then she asked me, 'What do you think about the idea of the toll gates?'

'What toll gates?'

'It is an old idea from the Church Fathers – that after you die the soul goes through a series of toll gates and at each one they are questioned and handed over to the demons to be punished before they can move on.'

I could feel the vomit rising in my throat, so I muttered something and put the phone down.

Those last hours with Deidre, the sense of love, of 'a place prepared for her' as Jesus had promised, had been one of the most precious experiences of my life. And now this person had suggested that after all she had already suffered, there was no such thing – only a series of torments on the soul's journey. Was this what I was supposed to believe? Not the experience of love?

Distraught, I dialled Father Richard's number and asked him if he knew about this. 'Don't worry about all that,' he told me. 'It's only projection on the part of some guy who has been sitting too long in the desert.'

The matron of the nursing home made me feel understood without ever saying anything explicit, and her kindness had been a real bridge between Deidre and me. She did not expect me to want to keep all of Deidre's things. In the end I took back two of her own (not very good) paintings of rural scenes, and a shoebox of photos and letters which I shoved to the back of a cupboard. I tried to hang up the paintings but could not, and put them up in the attic.

The next day I broke my foot stepping into the road in front of a cyclist. He was furious that I had ruined his trousers and I bought him a new pair. Even I realised I needed some time off, though I was worried about abandoning my clients without proper preparation. A therapist friend whose mother had died the year before recommended I took three weeks out as she had done. 'You'll find,' she told me, 'that your clients will survive. What they are really after is therapy, and they can live without you.'

She was right, and I needed the space. Grief began to give way to elation and a sense of freedom. It was spring, after all, and there were new ducklings on the river.

I began to dream about a baby girl, and took her to be a sign of new life in me. In the dreams she began to grow up until she was about three. Then she vanished. The last time I saw her, my mother and Nana were asking her to explain the meaning of 'Our Father...'

Part 4
INTO THE DEEP

1

Going Down

*I need a fix cos I'm going down – down to the
bits that I left up town*
The Beatles

For two years my horizon had been filled by Deidre, and suddenly I was free to get on with life again. 1999 was a good year. Then, on the Friday afternoon before Christmas I realised that something was seriously wrong.

It was not just the sense of dread: it was as though my whole body had been taken over. I felt sick and lethargic, and at the same time tense and wired up. By the time I started work again in the new year, it was as though a road block had been set up between me and my inner life. I was used to spending an hour alone every morning to read and reflect, but now I simply could not do that. Every time I sat down, my mind skittered off somewhere else. The only time I could make contact with my inner world was when I was working with clients, but that now exhausted me in a way that it never had before. I tried giving up caffeine to see if that would calm me down, but it made no difference. I tried, as I noted in my journal, 'to find some room in me for something other than survival'.

As for teaching, I wept all the way to work on Thursday mornings, and was terrified of breaking down in public.

Tears were followed by tears and more tears.

It was some while before I was ready to go and see Dr Gibson, my GP, because I knew she would prescribe anti-depressants. Though I would do anything to stop feeling like this, whenever I began thinking about taking any kind of drug I saw the drawer in my mother's kitchen: alongside the empty boxes of amphetamine and Tenuate Dospan (an alternative 'slimming pill') both of which had been declared Class 'A' drugs and taken out of circulation, there was Ritalin, Coproxamol, various sedatives and seven different varieties of anti-depressant: Prothiaden, Seroxat, Prozac, Gamanil ... . Each box was neatly labelled 'avoid alcohol'.

Then there was Pete and his terrible experience with Valium. All in all, it was hard to see drugs in a positive light.

Going back into therapy did not occur to me at first. I had had my three months with Mr O. and my five years with Patricia, as well as three years of group work in my training. That, I thought, was surely my ration. Increasingly desperate, I strayed into Holland and Barrett and bought a bottle of St John's Wort. It was, after all, a natural remedy, but even so I simply stared at the bottle of pills, too scared to take them.

After the half term trip to Cornwall with Jim, where I had the dream about having arranged for detectives to take my father away, spring arrived, but none of the things that normally gave me pleasure came anywhere near me. My forehead felt locked in a vice. Somehow I kept on working, but outside my consulting room if anyone asked me how I was I burst into tears. From time to time I felt a bit better. Then I would bump into someone I knew in the street and they would start to talk to me: any good feeling drained away like the bottom falling out of a bucket and I ended up staring at them in blank despair. Jim felt helpless and was in favour of me getting anti-depressants

Father Richard said he did not know what I could do except hope for it to pass. 'You have no choice but to endure,' he said, and it seemed to me possible that he felt a bit like this quite a lot of the time. 'But,' he added, 'the funny thing is that when you are tear-y, in a strange way it is not really you.'

I could not work out what he meant but it was somehow reassuring, as though there really was another me who was not like this.

Though I continued to see Andrew, my supervisor, about my work, it did not occur to me that my state of mind might be of interest to him. I did, however, phone Patricia and sobbed down the phone. 'What do you think about anti-depressants?' I asked her.

'In that state, I wouldn't hesitate', she said, 'There are loads of therapists who are only getting by on Prozac.'

But not me, surely?

Again I talked to Richard. 'I would recommend it', he told me, 'You drive yourself too hard'. He was not one to pull his punches. 'Perhaps,' he added, 'you need some humility about this.'

That hurt, but it also made sense. I was beginning to think that I needed to stop fighting the depression. I sensed there was something important about it, as though it was at last making me a member of the human race. Maybe I should start to acknowledge it, talk to it on its own terms.

A day or two later I phoned Richard and told him, 'I've made an appointment with the doctor, but I am still terrified of taking drugs.'

By now I could see he was in favour of them, but he was not going to push it against my will. 'The important thing,' he said, 'is that you keep control – as long as you are not damaging anyone else.'

He was right, as Patricia had been. It was not fair to my clients – or to my family – to ignore the state I was in. By not getting help for myself I was endangering other people. The next day I went to see Dr Gibson, and took the first pill.

I knew that Prozac took a week or two to kick in, but almost at once I stopped crying, though I was just as exhausted and still could not get my face to relax. The Prozac also churned up my stomach. 'Are you OK?' people kept asking. 'You look as though you need a good rest.' 'Look after yourself'.

Wondering what they saw, I gazed at myself in the mirror. To me I looked disappointingly all right so I asked Kathy what she thought, and she said I looked gaunt and tired, which was reassuring in a way. By now, something in me desperately wanted to be ill, wanted it all to be true. I wrote in my journal,

> *The depression has become my friend. It has become one of the most significant events of my adult life. I am no longer victimised by it. I am lying in it as in a bath, relaxed into it.*

Now that I had a diagnosis and a prescription I told Andrew that I had started Prozac. He was shocked to realise that I had got so low without telling him and said we would monitor how I got on. Being Andrew, he was also fascinated by my opportunity to see first-hand what the effects of the Prozac might be.

Something had to give, and I left my teaching job at the end of the spring term, just managing to make it through without phoning in sick. The students applauded my last lecture and as I walked out into the car park for the last time my colleague Toby ran after me with four glorious bunches of pink and red tulips.

So many people had given me things in the last few weeks: flowers, music, cards, even food. It was as though they all knew more than I did and were trying to look after me. The very next morning a client who had been seeing me about depression for several years walked in with another huge bunch of tulips, orange this time, and handed them over, saying cheerfully if a little defiantly, 'Spring!'

Meg was an artist and in spite of years of struggle with bipolar disorder she had always refused drugs, worried that they would interfere with her creative process. And here was I, the therapist, taking Prozac. *What would she say if she knew?*

One week into the Prozac, I had my first full night's sleep and began to tell myself life was not so bad after all. Kathy was thriving. She was able to sympathise with me without identifying, and she was revelling in the beauty of spring. Jim and I had a good enough life. Richard, Toby, Patricia and Andrew were all going on believing in me in spite of the depression. They had not abandoned me or written me off. This in itself felt as important as discovering I could recover from a miscarriage: I could be ill and depressed and not rejected. That made me think again about my mother and what she must have had to live with year after year. It made me very angry on her behalf.

I forced myself to think about what Richard had said about driving myself too hard. It was like running your tongue over a painful tooth, but I kept at it until I was able to consider it – and even to consider the possibility of being kind to myself, taking some real time off. After all, I had been working at my practice solidly for ten years and it would not be so terrible to take a break. I began to plan a two month sabbatical, to begin in August when most people would be away anyway. Even the thought of stopping work for a bit did me good. A day or two later I was amazed to find myself actually smiling, and although I still felt exhausted by lunchtime this was a great improvement on feeling exhausted all day.

Prozac was now my friend: an attack of diarrhoea sent me into a panic in case I had lost that day's dose. I refused to worry about getting dependent on it. This was short term treatment, I told myself, and Dr Gibson would monitor it carefully. She was not like the GP of one of my clients who had been issuing repeat prescriptions for Prozac for two years without ever seeing him. He wanted to come off it and was worried because a friend of his had killed himself soon after starting it. People had different reactions to it, I told myself firmly, and for me it seemed to be working.

After two weeks, there was a clear improvement: the stomach upset had settled and for a few hours each day I began to feel myself again. In between those times I still felt obscurely ill and none of it – even feeling ill – seemed quite real. The tension around my head went on. I slept at night now, but I was regularly overwhelmed by tiredness.

Because of the tiredness, Dr Gibson set up some tests for me at the hospital. The consultant said it was very unlikely but I might have TB, and he would send me an appointment for further investigations.

The next morning an envelope arrived from the hospital. *That's amazing,* I thought, *they must be really worried about me.* When I opened it there was a leaflet entitled 'Approaching death?' and I panicked. *So that is what he really thought.* It was only after a few moments that I realised it was nothing to do with my visit to the hospital but was from someone I supervised, advertising a conference she was setting up on death and dying.

Then, without warning, I started to go down again. Getting myself out of bed in the mornings was like peeling a sticking plaster off a wound, and I lost any sense that I might be recovering.

Clinically I knew this depression must be about loss and conflict. The reason I had no energy must be that it was all going to suppress something my conscious mind could not deal with. I could see there had been a lot of loss. A mother dying is a mother dying whatever the relationship has been like. And she had been the last of our parents' generation: Hugh, both my uncles and Hugh's sister Cordelia had all preceded her. By the time I was forty-six no-one but Pete remained from my original family. You may want to escape your family, but you do not expect them all just to curl up and die.

At last it occurred to me that I should get myself some therapy. I was ill, I said to myself, but I could get better, and therapy could help me. This was a reassuring thought, because to be depressed undermined my passionately held belief that to be like Deidre was unnecessary. I had always been determined that I could escape the sense of doom that surrounded her and fix up a good life for myself. On the whole so far I had managed that, and this was the first time I had found myself really losing control. If I could now accept that I was ill, however, and get help as I had done before with Mr O. and Patricia, I might be able to get better. Even the idea of getting help began to distance me from my mother, and made me feel less scared of turning into her.

Sleep had deserted me again and I lay awake at night thinking about her. Why had I always been so horrible to her? She had tried her best, but I had always been angry with her. In my efforts to love her I found myself angry with the whole idea of therapy. Therapy had enabled me to express my anger, and shed some of the guilt. But what about Deidre herself? Was there something about being a therapist, I wondered, that makes you so concerned to find the shadow side of people that you forget how to appreciate them in any ordinary way? Lying there in the dark, I tried to figure out what my mother's good points had been. Determination, loyalty to Uncle Jim, long term friendships. Those came easily enough. Tenderness? My imagination came to a stop there. I could not imagine Deidre being tender. Soggy, yes, but not tender. For as long as I could remember I had avoided touching her.

OK, what would be a natural reaction to your mother dying? A few days before Jim had said something about her and I had immediately been overwhelmed by waves of feeling I could not even name. Was that grief? I tried letting myself think about Deidre as you do with someone you miss, as I had seen other people think about their dead mothers, but I could not do it. Years before I had said to Mr O. that I could not imagine any situation that would be improved by my mother's presence.

'That is very sad,' he had commented, but in no way contradicted or judged what I had said. It was a simple fact. It would be crazy to pretend that I missed Deidre as other people missed their mothers, or even as I myself missed Hugh or Aunt Cordelia.

Whatever was going on, I decided, might be to do with my mother's death, but it went deeper even than grief. There was something inside me that was trying to get out, and my body and mind were doing everything they could to keep it down. Depression and repression are close allies.

For years I had wondered about there being some part of my story that I did not know about in spite of all the work I had done. Whenever I worked with people who recovered memories of abuse and accompanied them through that process, I wondered about myself. There were my vivid and violent dreams like the one about 'Russell Lockheart' which were becoming more rather than less frequent. There were shadowy attackers, absent rescuers, things about to happen that were so dreadful they could not be named. Then there were those seminars with Toby and the ordinands on sexual abuse when I would feel on the edge of panic. It was not that I was trying to avoid the truth. I had searched everything I could remember, but simply could not access any memory.

Then, along with sleeplessness, the nausea returned, and I was back to being constantly on edge. Periods – or rather premenstrual tension – became torture. It had always been a physical problem for me – feeling sore and bloated, and craving for chocolate – but now it was a mental one as well, hauling me to the brink of panic and hanging me over the abyss.

The first day that I was free from teaching, I finished printing out the final copy of a chapter I had written for a book on counselling edited by a colleague. It had been a struggle to write it but printing out the final draft should have been a moment of real satisfaction. Yet as each page came out of the printer and I laid it face down on the desk I was only aware of the page numbers getting bigger and bigger and this being some kind of threat. I found myself regarding each page as it emerged with dumb horror.

Perhaps this should not have been surprising. Most things felt like a threat at this time. I was constantly wide awake, and my face permanently tense. Even being with friends was difficult: it was as though I was behind a glass wall, cut off from what was going on around me. I had also come to dread the working day.

'I believe I will get through the day' I wrote in my journal. 'Seven clients. Seven nice people. I like them all. They like me. What am I afraid of?'

These were not, in fact, the easiest of sessions because I was now telling people about my plans for a two month sabbatical. One woman responded by sobbing for forty-five minutes of the fifty minute session. At the end of the afternoon I had to go to bed and fell into a deep sleep. When I woke up, I wrote to Mr O.

It was at this point that I decided to ask Dr Gibson for something to help me sleep. To me this meant I had given up, since I was even more terrified of sleeping pills than I was of anti-depressants: the thought that I would not be capable of waking up easily if something happened in the night was appalling to me. I may not have achieved the humility that Richard had recommended but I was giving up on my own self-image. That evening, I even went to the off licence and bought a bottle of whisky – Laphraoig single malt, but whisky all the same.

A large slug of it made no difference, and I was awake the rest of that night.

By morning I felt exhausted and wide awake. And mean. An acquaintance from church rang to ask if I would sponsor her on a walk to Iona in aid of something or other. *Why should I subsidise her holiday?* I thought, and told her I envied her doing the walk, and wouldn't be giving any money to it.

Dr Gibson produced a prescription for sleeping pills and I took the first one that night. It gave me a night's sleep and my psyche took the opportunity to produce a vivid dream:

I live in a hostel which is empty apart from one room occupied by me and a young man. The landlord lives seven miles away. One morning the landlord's daughter is found butchered – blood everywhere.

My roommate writes me a letter and tells me it was him. My first instinct is to keep quiet, but then I realise (a) that he committed a previous murder some years before and there might be others to come, and (b) the next victim might be me.

I go to the nearest town and manage to enlist two police women. (The male police are so busy they cannot do anything for two days, but I have left the murderer's letter in my room and need to get it back.)

> *The police women are driving me back to the hostel and saying it is quite safe because they are police. I say it is not safe because they are women and you can't argue with a psychopath.*

This dream – like so many others – had a 'no hiding place' quality: it may be possible to find some help, but the threat is greater than any help available. And I know more than is good for me.

The next day, a letter arrived from Mr O. He was willing to see me, and suggested I rang on Monday morning to make an appointment.

Life is good, I told myself. It is just that I am ill. But my friends don't abandon me. Neither did my mother's friends abandon her. Writing to Mr O. was the first step to getting my old self back.

It was strange then, perhaps, that I started forgetting to take the Prozac, and even forgot to phone Mr O. on the Monday morning as he had suggested.

Nevertheless, I began to feel a bit better. The sleeping pills worked, and it was wonderful to have some sleep now and then. Because they made me feel dopey in the mornings, I did not take them every night but only when I felt I could not go on any longer without sleep. One morning I lay in the bath and thought how difficult all that business with Deidre had been, and what a lot I had been through. No wonder I was battered by it. A thought wandered into my head: *Sometimes things get too much for me.* It was a delicious thought, and I thought it over and over again, like hugging a teddy bear.

A week later I rang Mr O. He sounded friendly and encouraging and we arranged to meet.

2

Searching

Why did I go to Mr O., and not to Patricia, or someone new? One reason was that any of the local therapists I knew and liked, including Patricia, I now knew far too well to work with them. Mr O. did not mix with our set, and our paths never crossed. Also, there were two pieces of unfinished business from our previous work, which lingered even after all this time.

The first was that I had once mentioned to a colleague that Mr O. was my first therapist. 'Oh yes,' she said, 'He is a marvellous person. I worked with him at the Clinic.' She knew about my religious interests and added, 'Did you know he was once an Anglican priest?'

I made some politely interested reply, but I was deeply shocked; it felt as though I had inadvertently told all my most intimate secrets to my father.

Then there was the remark Mr O. had made at the end of our last session, 'After all, you are a going concern.' Whenever I thought of that I felt cheated, dismissed. That feeling of mine reminded me of a phrase often used by Andrew, my supervisor, who was always keen to remember that healing is not necessarily about putting things back together, but also about letting them come apart. 'Sometimes,' he was fond of saying, 'you find there is something wanting or needing to break down'. Something in me quickened when Andrew said that, something that rebelled against being 'a going concern' and wanted to have it out with Mr O. Nobody, at least, could accuse me of being a going concern right now.

I also chose Mr O. because he was safe: a kind man who knew his boundaries and seemed unlikely to change. I also liked it that he always remained Mr ... and I Mrs... at a time when everyone seemed to have only first names.

He had retired from the clinic where I first saw him and had a small private practice at his house, where we sat in a cosy room with a fireplace and a grandfather clock. Our chairs faced the fireplace at an angle that made it easy to glance at each other, but did not require it. It occurred to me that I would have liked my father's study to be clean, tidy and cosy as this room was. How nice, I thought, it would have been if my father had been like this, always there to come back to, willing to listen, not dead of a heart attack at sixty-seven.... I wondered if Mr O. had daughters of his own and if they visited him here.

Much had happened since we worked together on the effects of my mother's miscarriage. There had been my own miscarriage, analysis, training, building my practice, my mother's death. Nevertheless, I began where we had left off twelve years before. 'Since I last saw you,' I said, 'I have thought a lot about something you said at the end of my last session, when you referred to me as "a going concern". It really affected me. That night, a friend came to supper and I poured a large gin and tonic and toasted myself: "Mr

O. thinks I am a going concern." It was a sort of joke, but I was angry. I felt kind of short changed.'

'You wanted someone to recognise that you might not always be a going concern?'

'Exactly'.

We agreed to meet for seven sessions. Why seven? I have no idea, but it is an interesting detail, given that the number seven kept turning up in my dreams: there would be a seven year old boy, or seven miles to go ....

I was still working, but it was a struggle. Slowly, steadily, my remaining energy was seeping away. I was intensely weary, and at the end of the working day would sink into bed and black out until Jim came home. I also found myself falling asleep – and occasionally dreaming – in sessions. It is not unheard of for therapists to fall asleep in sessions. I had a colleague who found herself regularly falling asleep with a particular client. Eventually she identified this as a powerful unconscious response – on her own part – to the fact that the client had spent a lot of her childhood sitting at the bedside of a sick mother. Again, one of my clients once remarked that he appreciated that I did not seem to find him boring. 'The last chap I saw,' he said, 'used to stand on his head in a corner of the room in order to keep awake.'

There was also the view expressed in an article by a Jungian analyst that falling asleep in the session was an excellent way of contacting the patient's unconscious, though I suspected he meant something a bit different from what was happening to me.

In other respects, I believed my work to be rather good at this stage since there was so little of me left that I was incapable of interfering with the other person's process. There may have been some truth in that. Amongst my colleagues there was a strong 'wounded healer' motif. We did not expect to be completely sane people in order to do our work. Rather we expected to be a little off *piste*: enough to be able to enter into a really mutual relationship with our clients – but not so much that we got swamped by it. I was not yet – quite – at the point where I had come apart so much that I was dangerous.

I often thought about a case study I had read of a little girl who was clever and good at school, but at home, when everyone was asleep, she went around the house hanging little bags of her own shit on all the door knobs. I could see that little girl. She was me. The school where she thrived was my prep school. The door knobs where I imagined her about her nightly work were the door knobs of our vicarage. By day I was still a just about good enough therapist, but by night I had more shit to deal with than I could handle. But now I had a space of my own, with Mr O.

My face felt as though it was locked in a vice. 'Why do I feel there is a knife down my throat?' I asked Mr O. 'Or that I have inhaled ground glass?'

I told him about family tea times in the vicarage. There would be a tea trolley in the sitting room with bread and butter, tea, cake, jam, and a few bone-handled tea knives. I regularly counted the knives, to make sure one of them had not gone missing. I needed to know because if it had, I thought I knew where it was – down my throat. Sometimes I would even get my mother to look down my throat to check if there was one there. She never saw one.

'You were a very vigilant child,' commented Mr O. He continued in that slightly humorous, questioning manner that a certain kind of therapist has. 'If you stop keeping watch for a moment, someone might stick a knife down your throat.'

We both laughed, and I felt hugely relieved. At last someone had recognised just how mad that child was – the child that was me.

The following week, however, he was shocked when I told him how good it had been to laugh. 'Did we really laugh?' he asked, shaking his head disapprovingly as though it really had been very callous of us.

He went on to muse about the knives, and what I might have been hoovering up from my mother's depression. 'She wanted you all dead,' he suggested. 'No room for a little girl.'

This was a fair comment considering the previous work we had done, but my unconscious was not going to let it rest there. That night I dreamed of a book with a blank page on which someone had written in large letters, 'IF YOU HAVEN'T GOT IT BY NOW …..'

The next day my bronchial tubes were burning, and by the weekend I recorded in my journal that my throat was on fire and my 'upper respiratory tract a sore mess'.

Since this showed no signs of going away, I went to see Dr Gibson and again I wept all over her office. She suggested signing me off for three weeks, and I wept even more. I could not abandon my clients. 'Are you fit to work now?' she asked gently.

'No,' I admitted, and she signed the paper.

There was no-one but me, of course, to ring and cancel all the sessions for the next two weeks. No-one but me to field the disappointment, anxiety and concern with which people responded to the news I was ill. I longed for a work place I could ring into, a receptionist who would cancel my appointments for me. Mr O.'s comment that I seemed to have to deal with everyone else's feelings before I could have my own was for a few days a practical reality – but finally I was free to sink into my own misery.

For months I had had a sense that I was approaching something I had been dreading all my life, what I described in my journal as a 'huge anxious feeling inside as though I'm about to go through a door.' Winnicott's insight, often quoted by Andrew in relation to my own clients, brought some comfort: 'Fear of breakdown is fear of a breakdown that has already happened'. This suggested that whatever was waiting for me, I had in some sense already survived it. I just hadn't managed to deal with it in my conscious mind.

When I did sleep, the pressure from the dream world was steadily building up. I kept dreaming about churches and there was one in particular that I kept going into. It was small, and it was down some steps. I was always anxious about losing the key. The church smelt of Brasso. I dreamed about murdered children, or children who were about to be murdered; about attacks and chases, and telephones that would not work; about child sacrifice in St George's. I dreamed of escaping with Nana across frozen wastes.

All I knew was, there had been an attack. Was it an attack on me, or on my parents, or on Pete?

There was also the repeated motif of the number seven. Why? My experience was that numbers in dreams are usually worth taking seriously. It was Kathy's seventh birthday that had triggered my journey into therapy, and it was a significant age in our family. My father had been sent away to boarding school at seven. My mother was seven when her father died. What had he really been like, and how had he treated his children?

Then there was my other grandfather, Hugh's father, whom I remembered only as a grumpy and self-important old man. My father's parents were wealthy but, according to my mother, 'They could never keep a maid because of Grandpa', so my aunt Cordelia had stayed home and skivvied for them until they died. My mother had even told me that when Hugh took her to meet his parents after they were engaged she was left alone with my grandfather in the dining room after lunch, and he started to fondle her breasts. She did not know what to do, she said, and was relieved when Hugh walked back into the room.

Maybe, I told myself, I was simply experiencing unprocessed family misery that had been passed onto me by some mysterious empathic process between generations.

What about the rising panic I felt in seminars on child sexual abuse? I had gone over and over in my mind the people I could remember from my childhood. Nothing. Our vicarage was on an island in the middle of a prosperous suburb. House, church and hall were on a patch of land surrounded by walls and hedges, beyond which were the streets. St George's loomed over our garden. We played in its shadow, shared its territory.

What about Mr Healey who always played the Wicked Uncle in the pantomimes, and lived with his mother? No. Little girls were in no danger from him. Or the organist? After all, I was seduced by my organ teacher when I was seventeen. Could it have been an echo of something earlier? I rang Pete because I could not remember anything about the organist at St George's. Analysis had put me in touch with a great many feelings, but as far as the facts of my childhood were concerned I was like a deaf-blind person: Pete was my eyes and ears.

'Do you know why I never sang in the church choir at St George's?', I asked him. 'It seems funny now I come to think of it.' After all, I had been insanely, painfully jealous of Pete serving in the sanctuary. I could have at least made it to the chancel.

'No, I don't. It does seem a bit odd now you mention it.'

'There was a choir, was there?'

'Oh yes. There was a choir of girls who all dressed up in cassocks and surplices.' He chuckled. 'You'd have liked that, dear.'

'Who played the organ?'

He thought a moment. 'That was Mr Woodman'

Mr Woodman. So it was. I could remember the name, and a lean, dark man.

'What was he like?'

'He was some sort of dark cloud as I remember. And he had a wife who suffered from nerves. She chain smoked and looked thin.' A vague image of a tense blonde floated across my internal field of vision.

'And there was Michael, the son. He played the drums in a pop group. I expect he's running a bank now. Except, no wait a minute, he married Jane Turner. I think he's a vicar.' Nothing there. It wasn't Mr Woodman, or his drum-playing son the vicar.

Who could tell me anything? Any other possible witnesses to an attack on me – parents, uncles, aunt – were all dead.

There was only Pete, but he was after all three years older than me. He might know something more. I rang him again. 'I need to talk to you. Can we meet up?'

'Of course. Do you want to come over here?' I did, but since by then I could hardly move from the sofa, he came to see me.

3

Attack

I don't know why nobody told you
how to unfold your love.
I don't know how
Someone controlled you
They bought and sold you...

The Beatles

IT WAS JUNE, an intense, stifling summer. I managed to make tea and get as far as the back garden where we sat opposite each other, Pete and I, in white plastic chairs. Behind him, drowsy flowers wilted in the heat.

I told him I had memories of an attack in childhood but I could not place it. 'I can't remember', I said, 'but everything tells me there was some sort of attack. And there is a lot about the number seven. Do you know something I don't?'

He did not answer right away, but something passed across his face. Then Pete – Pete the rebel, the drifter, the hard drinking, jazz playing, sixty-a-day-man truth teller; Pete who hated guys in suits, who went regularly to the brink of suicide rather than let a doctor foist Valium onto him – Pete turned clinical. 'I think', he said, 'we have to be so careful about memory. We never really know if we are right about it.'

He went back to London, and I to the sofa. Whatever he knew he was not going to tell me. And what he said was perfectly true: we do have to be careful about memory. It plays strange tricks. I decided that I should stop raking around inside myself and try to come to terms with grief for my mother and the rest of my family, in order to process whatever trauma I had inherited raw from the previous generation.

Accordingly, I explored the weight of our family history contained in the shoebox I had shoved to the back of a cupboard when my mother died. Mostly there were photos, on the back of which Deidre had scrawled names in red felt tip pen. My great grandmother, Hannah Brill, and her mother. A string of Nana's sisters: Flo, Eva, Lottie, Lill, all tough women. Some husbands, looking charming and a bit feckless. Holiday photos of people sitting on shingle like yogis on their beds of nails. A letter from Harry, Nana's brother, written from Allahabad in northern India on 13 September 1901, complaining that she had not sent him a photograph of herself:

> *Lill as been putting it off for about the same time and had the impotence to ask me for a silk kerchief but she has not got it yet and is not likely to before I get a decent photo not a penny one like she sent me some time ago … Flo says she had the offer of the place but refused it and recommended you. She must be very particular if a place that suits you will not suit her …*

With the letter was an *In Memoriam* card for Harry, killed on 31st January 1902 and buried at Allahabad. Also the Christmas and New Year cards Nana had sent him. She would have been fifteen years old, and already in service.

I tried to find a photograph of my mother I could bear to look at. There was the one of her as a child that had sat in our house with the glass cracked as long as I could remember. It gave me a cold feeling inside. There was a photograph of Hugh as a pantomime dame. I never had managed to keep photographs of my parents on display, though since the therapy with Patricia I had one or two of Nana. From time to time I tried to add Deidre and Hugh but the sight of them always made me feel so awful I put them away again. They gave me a feeling not so much of sadness or anger, as of bewilderment and an inability to be myself.

A therapist friend called by to see how I was and found me sifting through the photographs. 'You'll never be able to internalise them,' she remarked, 'They are such ambivalent objects.'

'You can't make a silk purse out of a sow's ear' said Mr O. at our next session. It would take years to understand what he meant. Now I just felt a desperate need to make amends for all the pain. I started by tracking down where my maternal grandfather had been buried in an unmarked pauper's grave. It only took a few phone calls. Deidre had wanted his name included on her tombstone. Now, I thought I could visit the actual place, maybe even erect a stone, but I did not have the energy. It was only up the road from where we had lived in London, and it did occur to me to wonder why she had not done this herself.

I still expected to return to work at the end of the two weeks of being signed off. In spite of my anger with Mr O, I was determined to be a going concern, even with apparently permanent flu and a raging sore throat and chest. All I needed was to let go of the past. 'I've had four of the seven sessions with Mr O.,' I told Richard, 'and I think the remaining three will be enough. I can feel my life beckoning, present and future, and I want to live it.'

Then, nine days after his first visit, Pete came again, this time at his own suggestion. In the intervening time he had been to see his therapist, to ask, 'Should I tell her?'

For five years, he had been asking her this question, and she had always said, 'Not so long as she is functioning OK'. Now it was different. 'She deserves to know,' she had said at last.

Again I made tea for Pete and myself, but although it was still hot outside it seemed right to stay indoors, huddled in armchairs in the dark Victorian sitting room. What we had to talk about did not belong in the sunshine. I said again that I had a sense of an attack, that my nightmares suggested something happening when I was about seven.

There was a pause, and then Pete asked, 'Have you ever wondered about Perks?'

Perks. The wrinkled man in the dark grey suit with black rimmed glasses and a scar on his cheek. Occasionally in recent months, as I surfaced from yet another nightmare, his name had wandered into my head. Sometimes even his face, with the glasses and the scar. Had I wondered about him? No, though I had once or twice allowed half a thought to surface and then dismissed it.

Perks, Phil Perkins, was a full time paid verger at St George's. He swept the floors, polished the brass, stoked the boiler, put out the dead flowers. He also wound the large and scary clock, whose mechanism ticked and creaked in a glass fronted cupboard at the back of the nave. At Christmas he decorated the big tree, having amongst his treasures some shiny feathery birds which I loved. Some mornings he came in early to answer the Mass said daily by my father before breakfast. Every day at noon he would ring the *Angelus.*

'Mum, what does "Hour of our death" mean?'

'It's from the Hail Mary. "Hail Mary, full of grace ..."'

'Perks?', I asked myself again as I sat there with Pete. No, that was ridiculous. I could never have been attracted to Perks.

' ... the crypt,' I heard Pete say.

'What crypt?'

'You know, the crypt where John Ward lived.'

Right now I could not get my mind to picture a crypt, though I had to accept that it existed, because rationally I knew that what Pete was saying was true, that for a while our father had let a man live − or rather camp − down there.

'I think John was all right,' Pete went on. 'I was fascinated by him, and went to see him a lot, but I don't think there was anything funny about him. He was a message from another wavelength − modern, socialist and all that.'

Something shifted in my memory. 'He had a motorbike,' I added. Like Pete, I liked that 'outside' character that Other People like John had, people who were not part of the church. Our Uncle Paddy, Deidre's brother, was another one. 'I suppose Paddy was also a message from the outside world.'

'Yeah' said Pete, 'Though Paddy was cheery like Herman Goering, that jolly old Nazi. What a weird world.'

The crypt, Pete went on to remind me, was part of Perks's territory, along with the vestry and the boiler room.

'Where was it?' I asked finally, feeling stupid. I had played over this territory for the first twelve years of my life, but my mind *would not* go there. 'The crypt, that is.'

'You know – round the back, where the church joins onto the hall. You went past the boiler room, and down a few steps.'

'Still can't see it.' Though I was beginning to get the boiler. A black door open onto flames that Perks fed with his shovel. The gaping mouth of hell.

'Perks was always threatening to put me in that boiler,' mused Pete.

We had a coke boiler in our kitchen, too, a much smaller one of course. It had a little round lid which was lifted up with a metal tool, and then let drop. I remembered, time after time, hearing the sound of that lid dropping, screaming, and racing to the kitchen to check that Timmy, my little pink teddy bear, had not been put inside. As Mr O. had pointed out, I was a very vigilant child.

'But what happened to you' Pete said, 'wasn't when you were seven. It was much earlier.' He paused. 'Did you know,' he asked, 'about Perks dying of cancer while you were away in Canada? It must have been the 70s.' It was when I was in Canada that I had the dream about the replica of St George's on Vancouver Island which gave me a panic attack. *No, it's just a clever replica – a tourist attraction. St George's really is in England.'* ... *'You must paint this out. It's the only way you'll ever get over it.'*

'No,' I said to Pete. 'I didn't know anything about Perks dying.'

'Well, Deidre and Hugh kept in touch with him after they moved and he retired. And when he got cancer they used to go over to sit by his deathbed. It was quite a long journey. Anyway, I was there one day when they came back and Deidre started telling me how he was in all this awful pain and they could do nothing about it. "That's terrible," I said. And she answered, "No it's not. It's great. I sit there and relish every moment of it after what he did to Carolyn."'

What?

'What?' I asked eventually. Pete went on. 'It was when you were quite small. You went over to the church one day and you came home very distressed. You wouldn't speak. And there was white stuff in your knickers. She was very confused by that – and so was I. After all, semen wouldn't be white by the time it had dried, would it.'

Words came from somewhere not myself, and used my mouth to be spoken. 'No. He had his penis in my mouth and his hand in my knickers.'

We waited together in silence as they sank in.

Then Pete continued with some of his Perks-related reminiscences. There was the time Pete found a monkey wrench lying on the garden path and hit Perks with it so hard he drew blood. Our father beat him for that. 'He did the whole formal public school thing: bend over, shake hands afterwards. I suppose he had to do it sometime.'

He also told me how for years before our mother died she used to call on him every week on her way back from Uncle Jimmy's and talk endlessly about what Perks had done to me.

'She used to go on and on about it, especially after Hugh died. She'd bring a bottle of Scotch and by the time it was half empty we'd had it all. You, and Perks, and how it had wrecked your life. You seemed pretty OK to me. You'd managed to escape from Her, anyway.' It had worried him, though – hence the discussions with his own therapist.

'We have a shared history,' he said finally, 'and it nearly killed me, and there is no way I would inflict it on anyone. But at least I can say I've been an alcoholic and a drug addict and suicidal, dropped out of university and all that, whereas you – you've kept going, and in a way that's worse.'

The whole world turned upside down. Perhaps it was not so strange after all that I resented being a going concern.

As soon as Pete left, I rang Richard, and yes he was in, and yes I could go and talk to him. He listened to me. He believed me. He said what a marvellous brother I had. I noticed his comment and did not react. Again, it took years to sink in just what Pete had done for me. I was used to being the one who worried about him, not the other way round.

4

The Scene of the Crime

ON SUNDAY, I went along to the morning Eucharist as usual. I was pleased to see that the first hymn was an ancient Latin one about the completion of the salvation story as something here and now, already achieved and assured.

Christ is made the sure foundation, And the precious cornerstone, Who, the two walls underlying, Bound in each binds both in one ...

The organ played over the first couple of lines, and I opened my mouth to sing. Nothing happened. I tried again. It was simply impossible to make any kind of sound. Every time I tried I felt as though I was choking. Quietly I put the book down on the chair next to me and moved to an empty corner at the back of the church where I could sit with my eyes closed, letting the service carry on around me. I felt very safe and protected there, and did not move, even to go to communion. As I left a young woman who had been there with her small children came up to me. 'You are ill,' she said. 'Believe me, I know about these things, and you are very ill.'

She did not ask anything, and I did not want her to, but it helped. She had named something I could not quite take in for myself.

For the rest of that day I stayed home. My body was taken up with remembering things: the rape in my mouth, a terrible experience of being shaken, pain. That night I was woken by some kind of convulsion.

In the morning I was due for a session of cranial osteopathy which I had begun earlier in the year, because the symptoms of the depression were so physical and I hoped it might help re-align the energies that had deserted me. Once a month I lay on a couch in a quiet room smelling of herbs and a woman called Lydia laid hands on different parts of me. We did not talk about my state of mind, but I could tell that her hands were listening to my body and normally I found this very soothing. Today I was terrified of what her hands might hear.

'Have you had a shock in the last few days?' Lydia asked after I had lain there for a while.

'I suppose – yes – a bit of one'. I did not want to talk about it and said nothing more.

'I'm going to give you some Rescue Remedy', said Lydia at the end of the session. 'There is a scream being held in your body from the bladder upwards.' She did not ask for details – they belonged with Mr O. – but she did prescribe me some herbal mixture. When I got home I began to shake all over.

After what seemed a long time, it was the day of my appointment with Mr O., and I was able to tell him what Pete had told me. I do not know what I expected but I was vaguely surprised that he took the story seriously, and even added some thoughts based on what we had talked about before – the anxiety about a knife down my throat, the feeling as though I had swallowed ground glass.

161

'You may well have had a knife *to* your throat,' said Mr O. 'Or did he threaten to throw you in the boiler if you told anyone?'

Come on, my mind was saying. *Isn't this a bit dramatic? This is Perks we are talking about. Me. St George's. Isn't this guy a bit over the top? Bloody therapists.*

Then questions began to flood in. Did it happen the summer before I started school? I was four in May that year. Was that why I refused to speak for the whole first term? Was I scared of saying the wrong thing to the wrong person and ending up in the church boiler? And why was I so scared they would throw Timmy my pink teddy bear into the kitchen boiler? Was it some kind of substitution? If I was four that year, Pete would have been seven ...

Still I said nothing to Jim. I could not yet bear to talk with a sexual partner about what had happened.

As for Richard, I knew he had been wonderful the day Pete came, a priest who – unlike my father – had heard me, believed me, and listened compassionately. Yet suddenly I was terrified of him, feeling completely cast out and alienated. All I could think was that he must surely be disgusted with me now. As a therapist I knew that I must have transferred to him feelings I had as a child after the event, probably towards my father. But as with all transference, they were real feelings. Then he rang, having noticed that I had not come to communion at the Eucharist a few days before. I did not know what to say, and there was a short silence. 'What's up?' he asked, nonchalantly.

I knew I had to check whether what I was feeling was real – whether it was mine or his – and told him about it.

'It feels,' I finished up, 'as though now you know what

you do about me you won't want any more do with me.'

Richard did not hesitate, and his reply was simple. 'I feel rather hurt that you could think that of me.'

Until that moment it had not occurred to me that Richard had emotions and could express them. But what he had said was fine. I was not terrified of him anymore. He mentioned he had a meeting in London in a few days and I asked him if he would do something for me: he agreed. We arranged that I would go with him in his car to London and wait while he went to the meeting. Then he would take me to see St George's, the place where I grew up.

There it all was, looking just as it had in another life. Richard parked outside the vicarage and we walked around the perimeter wall to see the church. There was the porch where we used to sing Christmas carols around the tree. I stood looking at it for quite some time.

'Where's this crypt then?' asked Richard as though it was the most natural thing in the world. I could still barely believe it existed, but we walked on around the church, past the parish hall. There at the back of the church was the boiler house, and steps down to a white door. The crypt. The same small 'church' down some steps, with a smell of Brasso, that I had been dreaming about. Perks' territory that had been wiped from my mind for forty-four years.

My three weeks' sick leave was almost at an end, and I still thought I could go back to work until the end of July when my sabbatical was due to start. After that I would have time to take stock. I'd accessed the story, visited the scene of the crime. Now I could put it all on hold for a few weeks. After all, I thought, I could not just walk out on all these people – and yet I had to admit I did not want to see them, and felt bad about this. I found that I also resented the thought of being a 'going concern' even for a few weeks

'I've been feeling a kind of resentment,' I told Richard as we drove up the motorway, 'against the people I see for therapy because it was so hard to keep going all through the two years leading up to my mother dying and even more so for the last six months. But that is not their fault! And what has happened now is not their fault either.'

He did not reply.

Back home, the anti-therapy feelings I had had early on with Patricia came back more strongly than ever. Everything about therapy infuriated me: people having to pay for help, all these boundaries, the dull, sensible 'parenting' I received from Mr O. – and gave as a therapist. The whole therapy enterprise, I told myself, was in denial, pretending that all you needed was to set boundaries and everything would fall into place. What nonsense! Life was shit and life was chaos: no pretence at making it manageable could set this to rights. At that moment I *needed* chaos, just as I had needed the rusty cars on the Indian Reservation, and the crazy disorder of Jim's office.

Fortunately, I had supervision with Andrew that week and told him what had happened. He helped me to understand I could not go back to work. With his help, I managed to find other people to take on my clients, made the necessary phone calls and wrote the necessary letters.

Andrew did everything anyone could. He had been a good 'father' to me throughout the time I had been working as a therapist. Now I was losing him too, since without a practice I no longer needed a supervisor.

'You have another job to do now,' Andrew told me as I

left his room for the last time.

I was devastated. It had taken ten years to build that practice and I could not believe I was abandoning it, even though everyone gently explained to me that it would be unethical to continue. Worse, I felt like a pariah: unclean, and unfit to be a therapist. With this came a terrible sense of shame.

'You don't require anyone to judge you,' remarked Mr O. when I told him about this at our next session 'It's all there inside you.'

At last I was free now to do what Andrew had called my 'other job.' Free to lie on the floor playing *Abbey Road* and the *White Album* over and over again: *Once there was a way to get back homeward. Once there was a way to get back home …*

Even I accepted I had to go on with Mr O. beyond the original seven sessions. 'I don't want to,' I wrote in my journal, 'but I feel I must. All I *want* is to be loved back to life by my real friends.'

Meanwhile, I stopped taking Prozac. Taking it made me angry, as though I was a child being given sweets to stop her crying. This was no longer about me having a depression, but about something that had been done to me. As I noted in my journal, 'I don't feel clinically depressed, only in a state of shock, grief and raw anger.'

I asked Richard if he thought it was safe to come to communion in this state. I wanted to, but to me communion was darkness and fire as well as acceptance and healing, so I was anxious about mixing it with my internal state. Richard's reply was extremely gentle. 'If you are going to,' he said, 'you have to think of yourself like the man that was found by the Good Samaritan, who had been beaten by thieves – and of communion as the wine and oil poured into the wound.'

The following week I paid another visit to St George's, this time with Pete, and we went inside the church. It looked much the same as it used to, except that the high altar was no longer in use, and there was a table at the bottom of the chancel steps. The bell rope where Perks used to ring the *Angelus* still hung to one side.

Then we walked around to the crypt and tried the door. It was locked. Finally, we rang the doorbell of the vicarage. A woman answered.

'Is the vicar in?' I asked.

'No, but I am the parish administrator,' she said, 'Can I help?'

'My brother and I', I said, 'lived here years ago, when our father was vicar. Our parents have died recently, and we wondered if we could have a look around. It's just part of the grieving process.'

'Well I'm afraid the vicar's not here,' she replied, 'but you can come into the office.'

The office was Hugh's old study. It no longer needed tidying up, and there was no knee-hole desk. The armchairs either side of the fireplace where we had sat for my Latin lessons had been replaced by tables, which had papers and files stacked on them.

'Do you think the vicar would mind if we had a look at the garden?' I asked, adding as casually as Winnie-the-Pooh on a bad day, 'And is there a key for the crypt?'

She gave us the key, and off we went. I was expecting to see the shelves with Brasso, the flower vases, the figures and straw for the crib and the feathery birds for the Christmas tree: all the things I had loved to help Perks with. They had all gone. The crypt was now a chapel for children.

Afterwards we walked across to the vicarage garden, which had hardly changed. It was broad and gracious, with flower beds up against the bay window. As we stood on the lawn, gazing out over the high brick wall to the rooftops across the road, Pete had a sudden panic attack. I put my arms around him. 'What is it?' I asked, holding him.

He wept. 'It's standing here, and looking Out There', he said, sobbing. 'All those places I didn't want to go. The "real world", school, all that.'

We went back and dropped the key through the vicarage letter box. I never would understand what it was that made Pete want to stay at home.

Part 5
AFTERMATH

1

Unexploded Bomb

THERE WERE SO MANY THOUGHTS in my head that I was glad no words were required next time I lay down on Lydia's couch.

'Do you mind if I work on your head today?'

'Fine.'

She settled herself on a stool behind me and took my head in her hands. 'Is that all right for you?'

'Yes'

'Not too much?'

I did not bother to answer. I had no way of telling whether a thing was too much or not. With my head in her hands like that, she must know everything I was thinking anyway.

After a while she asked, 'Have you ever had a bang on the back of the head?'

'Why?'

'There is something here like an old, old bruise. It is as though you are trying to repel something unpleasant from your mouth.'

My breath seemed to get stuck half way up my chest. After a moment or two I replied in my best clinical manner, 'I think you are dealing with an oral rape at the age of four.'

This made sense to her. She explained that the hippocampus, where long term memory is formed, is still undeveloped at that age: only the body can remember. My head, she remarked, was like an unexploded bomb.

In the weeks and months that followed I hung on to what Lydia had said because I still found it difficult to believe the words that had come out of my mouth that day with Pete. Mr O. believed it, Richard believed it, Andrew believed it, and Patricia, as did the friends I told. Mr O. said an exquisite thing that I could hardly take in. 'It must be very difficult to discover something like this at this point in your life.'

I went over and over that sentence in my mind. From a great distance I could see what was contained in it. He had not only told me he believed me, but he had also responded to me as a colleague – a real person with a real life. But my mind always skidded off into bewilderment when I tried to think about that.

One of the people I told was Toby, the colleague who had given me flowers on my last day of teaching. He took me in his arms and said, 'That makes sense. There was always a kind of deadness about you when I hugged you.'

It was a strange kind of affirmation – brutal, but acknowledging the problem. I told him about the feelings I had as though I had been shaken, and he asked, 'Are you sure there is not something to do with your father?'

Yes, I was. It seemed unimaginable that he should even think it possible. Then again, I was not certain of anything anymore.

There were several men looking after me – Mr O., Richard, Andrew, Toby, Pete – but I barely spoke to Jim about what was going on. He knew I was ill, and he knew what had happened, but we did not discuss it. When I did eventually tell him about the conversation with Pete the best he could manage was, 'Well, you have to understand these things happen.'

As often happens the person closest to me was the least able to support me. My discovery was an invasion of his world too. When he was around in the evenings, I did my best to behave as though everything was normal. It was during the long empty days, in my dreams, and while lying awake at night that I hung my metaphorical parcels of shit on the doorknobs.

Although as a therapist I had accompanied other people on similar journeys to mine, I found it hard to hang on to the self who had been able to do that, or to apply the same level of understanding to myself. I went over and over my text books on sexual abuse, needing someone or something to confirm that everything I was feeling was perfectly normal for a 'survivor'. Well, as Pete and Mr O. had both pointed out, I'd always been one of those – except I didn't feel much like surviving these days.

'Intense affective reactions to the recovery of memory of sexual abuse may be accompanied by self-destructive behaviours, e.g. suicide attempts.'

I had known that for a long time and seen it happening: now I understood it from the inside. I had lost all sense of my own worth, to myself or anyone else. Kathy was fine now, I told myself, living her own life. She might grieve a bit if I died, but she would get over it. I would leave her a letter telling her how much I loved her. As for Jim, he would probably be relieved. He had cried for a week when his mother died, and then never mentioned her again. Probably it would be the same with me, and he would soon find someone new.

It was nearly twenty years since I had given up smoking. Now I began again, inhaling viciously and relishing the damage I was doing to myself. The books were onto this, too: a return to old addictive behaviours was common in the first months after disclosure, they said, and not to worry too much: the desire would pass. It would be five years before I managed to kick the habit again. I lay on the floor of what had been my consulting room with an ashtray beside me, filling the air with smoke while the Beatles held my brain and prevented it from shattering into pieces.

I'm so tired, I'm feeling so upset.

Because I'm so tired, I'll have another cigarette.

And curse Sir Walter Raleigh, he was such a stupid get …

One reason I needed the books to tell me that all this was normal was that I could not get over the feeling that I had no right to feel this bad, that I was malingering. Maybe I had made the whole thing up because I wanted an excuse for a holiday?

Nobody was questioning the truth of what I had said – but then they, too, had read the books. They, too, knew that you should never disbelieve a first disclosure, and should show 'calm concern without disgust'. There was no doubt that that was what they had done, but maybe they were humouring me. Maybe they secretly knew I was mad, and were waiting their chance to get me into hospital.

There were days when I lay in bed and fantasised that I *was* in hospital, in a quiet, clean room where I was allowed to sleep all day. In my fantasy, Richard would come to visit, and the nurse would tell him in hushed tones that he could sit beside me so long as he did not disturb me. Then he would come and sit by my bed for a while before very quietly getting up and leaving. It was very soothing.

Another couple of weeks passed and I was due to go for a few days to a cottage in the Normandy countryside with Aileen, an old friend from before I became interested in therapy. This trip belonged amongst the shreds of normality that remained and it did not occur to me that spending a week with me in my current state of health might prove a severe test of friendship. I was still refusing to take Prozac, though Kathy persuaded me it would be a good idea to take it with me to France in case I needed it. Aileen came to stay the night before we left. We sat at the kitchen table having tea, and she commented, 'You've become a monster smoker all of a sudden. What's happened?'

I told her, and she responded with a matter of fact sympathy.

The cottage was a long, low building a mile or so from a walled village. From the sitting room a corridor led back to two bedrooms, with a bathroom at the end. We arrived in the late evening, and went to bed.

My room was clean and bare, with a single bed, a table, a wardrobe and a wooden chair. It was just the kind of room I might have had in the hospital of my fantasy. The journey had exhausted me and I quickly fell deeply asleep.

It was still dark when I found myself coming up out of sleep, screaming – or trying to. My mouth and nose were stuffed with something that refused to give way, something unmentionable. As soon as I was fully awake it vanished and I could breathe again.

Outside there were no cars, no street lights. Nor was there a bedside lamp, but I did not mind because I knew that I was safe here in my little room as long as I lay absolutely still in the dark and the silence. Even to reach out and put on a light would have disturbed the stillness and I stayed exactly where I was under the covers. It felt as though something was nourishing me, and whatever it was reminded me of James Naylor, a seventeenth century Quaker who was tortured and imprisoned. His account forms part of the Quaker tapestry:

> *There is a Spirit which I feel that delights to do no evil nor to revenge any wrong, but delights to endure all things in hope to enjoy its own in the end … if it be betrayed it bears it, for its ground and spring is the mercies and forgiveness of God. Its crown is meekness, its life is everlasting love unfeigned, it takes its kingdom with entreaty and not with contention, and keeps it by lowliness of mind. I found it alone, being forsaken.*

I found it alone, being forsaken. For me that summed up everything I believed in. Even though I was so angry about being myself a forsaken, raped child, I now believed, as a matter of experience, that love existed. All would be well, so long as I could stay exactly where I was, not moving, alone in the dark.

It was then that I noticed the pressure on my bladder, and realised what was required of me: to get out of bed, cross the room in the dark to the light switch, go out into the hall and find my way to the bathroom. You might as well have asked me to walk into a lion's cage. Slowly, I forced my mind to study the facts. It was the year 2000. We were in France. There was nothing in the room and nothing outside it except the countryside. Finally I reminded myself that a few yards away, in her room across the hall, Aileen was sleeping. Because she was there, I could do it.

We had planned to revisit walks we had enjoyed on a previous visit but on the first attempt my body simply gave up. I collapsed and sat by the roadside unable to move, and Aileen had to go back for the car to collect me. Back in the cottage, I retired to the sofa in the living room. Aileen let me sleep for a while, then brought in a cup of tea, sat on the end of the sofa, and gently tried to persuade me that maybe it might be a good thing to restart the Prozac. She knew about Prozac. As a teacher she regularly took it in term time, and came off it during the holidays.

'But do you believe me, about what happened?' I asked.

'Of course I do,' she said.

'But I've no real evidence. Maybe I made it all up.'

'Why would you do a thing like that?'

With Aileen's help I started Prozac again. There was the usual acidic feeling in my stomach for the first few days, but it no longer felt like sweets being given to a child to shut her up. It was going to help me get well.

A day or two later, I asked Aileen again if she believed me. She sat me down, put her hands on my shoulders and looked me in the eye. 'Listen,' she said, 'You have been horribly betrayed.'

Her word, 'betrayed', caught my attention. It was not one I would have thought of myself. Now Aileen had used it I realised that she meant that people whom I should have been able to trust to care for me had not done it.

Not everyone would have lasted the week with me, but Aileen did.

Back home, I began to believe myself at last. But so what if it *was* true? I had worked with people whose stories were far worse than mine: children who had been repeatedly raped by their fathers; children who had spent years in terror of the next door neighbour, uncle, older brother, stepmother; children who had been threatened with all sorts of things if they ever dared to tell. Well, I supposed I could chalk up that one: the school term when I had not spoken, and the panic about the kitchen boiler and my teddy bear.

The small scale of my story did not seem to bother other people. When I tried out my trivia theory on Richard. He frowned in a puzzled kind of way and said, 'This kind of thing is like an earthquake'.

One day I went back to see Andrew, my supervisor, to bring him up to date. Towards the end of our session, I mentioned that I had a great longing to sit with Meg, my client who was an artist and who had once brought me flowers to celebrate spring. My relationship with Meg had always embodied what my colleagues and I meant by mutuality. Although she could be very fragile emotionally, there was something in her that was deep and strong and nurturing. Our mothers had died around the same time – hers much loved – and when mine died and I took some time out she coped well with the unexpected separation and wrote me a wonderful letter. At the time when I became ill we had begun to talk about ending, and when I

175

stopped working she chose not to see anyone else.

A year or two earlier I had been to an exhibition of her work held in her house and caught sight of her small, clean, old fashioned kitchen with its scrubbed table and neat dresser. Now I longed to sit with her in that kitchen. Andrew smiled and said, 'Why don't you write to her?'

I did write to Meg, and went back to blocking my ears with the Beatles:

Blackbird singing in the dead of night, take these sunken eyes and learn to see. All your life, you were only waiting for this moment to be free.

On some level I believed this, even now.

The person I thought about most was my father, and the feelings of terror and alienation I had about Richard when I first remembered the rape. Interpreting those feelings as transference, they must relate to how I had experienced my father at the time. Had he been disgusted by me – rather than by what had happened to me? Or did he even know? Pete had not mentioned whether Hugh knew anything. Had I been over-sexualised in my approach to him, and experienced some terrible rejection?

My feelings for Hugh had always been confused. People often said how close we were, and we certainly were alike in many ways. Although I never really knew what he was thinking or feeling, his presence was comforting. Yet we had not spent any time alone together since my teens – and I had, of course, rejected the church – the very thing that was at the centre of his life. We never talked about that, but I was constantly aware of it and the guilt that followed from it. I could also be quite cruel. The last time I saw him before he died I deliberately told him that I had gone out with a friend and our small children to the zoo on what had been Maundy Thursday. I saw a look pass over his face, but he did not say anything.

While in therapy with Patricia, I had had a vivid dream in which I was a child and simply adored my father. The dream was full of light. Now I remembered Freud saying that at the root of melancholia there can be anger with someone one ought to love. Was being angry with my father at the root of my depression? It was true that my feelings for him now oscillated between rage (which hurt because I longed to love him) and a terrible desire to accept his verdict against me and whatever punishment might go with it. I found myself longing to be obliterated, and searched inside myself for something to counteract that.

'What are you angry with your father about?' asked Mr O., but I had no answer to that.

There was a curate at my church who had a four year old daughter, Susie, and I found myself watching her with him, trying to imagine what it might have been like to be me before the rape.

I also went back to *The Tempest* – to Prospero and Miranda. Like them, we had lived on an island, the island of St George's. Like them, we had a Caliban – but my father had not been a Prospero. He had not said to Perks, 'I did treat thee, filth, as human, and shared my cell with thee, until thou didst seek to violate the honour of my child.' He had gone on employing him, and even visited him on his deathbed. When I had thought about that for a bit, I wrote him a letter, struggling to speak as one adult to another:

.... Whatever went on between us back then felt to me

177

like a punishment that went so deep that I had to struggle to find my right to exist. Part of me longs to accept your verdict because to me you were perfection. My Daddy. But I also know that it's not going to help either of us if I allow myself to be obliterated.

For little Susie, her Daddy is everything. You can hear the delight in her voice when she shouts 'Daddy!' and rushes for his black cassocked legs ... I am sure I felt the same way about you. But I didn't know my boundaries, my beginnings and ends, or who belonged where, because of what happened to me.

This was too hard for you. What I experienced as your disgust with me was your own disgust with yourself ... two confused, damaged people frightened by the erotic power of love ... We lost so much ... We never quite loved each other freely again ...

What Perks did, he did to the whole family.

That was one way of looking at it. Yet, when I thought about my parents, I could not see them simply as fellow victims. They both knew, and they had said nothing to me. They had even died knowing and not telling me. Pete knew. Even Pete's therapist knew. Everyone knew except me. And my parents had been in touch with Perks until he died, years later. OK, my mother's attitude to the deathbed visiting was a little unusual for a vicar's wife, but they had visited with him, and had *appeared* solicitous. How could they? How dare they?

'Wouldn't it make someone angry,' I asked Richard, 'if someone did what Perks did to their daughter?'

Richard did not hesitate. 'That,' he said, 'is the kind of

thing people commit murder for – in any civilised country.'

OK. But my father hadn't murdered anyone. He had even beaten Pete for attacking Perks with the monkey wrench.

Well, it was a different generation, and I was used to the many forms of denial practised by the parents of abused children, having heard a great deal about them in my work.

Slowly, however, I began to confront the thing I dreaded, the thing the bishop had said at my father's funeral, about his love for the Eucharist, the 'table that he loved', the altar. It was a table that I now also loved, and being accepted at it week by week was one of the things that was holding me together. However disgusted I might feel with myself, I was still able to receive the bread and the cup with the other members of the congregation, and each time I felt flooded with gratitude for that acceptance.

After that long ago day when I had 'come home very distressed' my father had gone on ministering at that table – and part of Perks' job was to answer early morning Mass. It was as though I had a knife in my gut and was bleeding all over the carpet.

The phone rang and it was Meg, my client, responding to my letter. 'Do you realise I haven't seen you for six and a half weeks?' she asked.

No I didn't. It did not seem possible. For years my life had been governed by the weekly rhythms of therapy. Meg and I had worked for several years with the minutiae of the gap between one Friday and the next. It was shocking to realise that that six and a half weeks had gone by without my noticing it. I had simply been in limbo.

I did go and see Meg, and sat in her peaceful kitchen. I explained what had happened and she was kind to me; at the same time she was able to tell me how she felt about me abandoning her and I managed to survive that. It took time, but we developed a deep and lasting friendship.

Meanwhile, it was coming up to Mr O.'s summer break. I felt very low about that and now became obsessed with guilt about the people I had let down when I closed my practice. How could I have done this to them? Was I giving my clients an angry message by refusing to see them, I asked him.

'No,' Mr O. reminded me. 'Objectively you can't do it.'

That afternoon I rang Andrew and he repeated the same answer. Still unconvinced, I rang Patricia and asked her whether by closing my practice I was passing on the abuse, the neglect that I had experienced, to my clients. 'No,' she replied gently, 'You are not abusing them, honey.'

Having heard them all, I was overtaken by lethargy.

'I am aware of being angry,' I wrote in my journal, 'in the same way I am aware that the sun is shining.'

Guilt was now the biggest thing on my horizon, and driven by a need for atonement I volunteered for the church cleaning rota. I desperately wanted to serve the church, just as I had once desperately wanted to be kind to Corinna and give her the last piece of toast after I realised she was sleeping with Susanna Taylor. Once a week I went in and polished the brass. There was something strangely comforting about smell of Brasso. I must have liked pottering around with Perks, just as I liked his stores of vases, cleaning materials and Christmas decorations in the crypt. All these belonged to a world in which the rape had not happened. I could see the inside of the crypt now: a long, low room with whitewashed walls, and old wooden white painted shelves running down one side. *There was white stuff in your knickers...* Damp, flaky white walls. White stuff in my hair. White stuff on Perks's hands ...

At last, my throat and chest were returning to normal, but I had a new problem which was to plague me for more than a year to come. I thought of it as 'the thing in my mouth' and it is best described as a kind of fart: a build-up of something in the roof of my mouth which could only be released by something between a croak and a belch. Over time, it gradually worked its way from the back of my throat into the roof of my mouth to behind my front teeth. I had no control over it, and if I was tired it went on almost continuously, like a bad attack of wind. My doctor called it *globus hystericus.* There was no treatment, and only cigarettes soothed it.

In early September the principal of the college where I had taught came to see me, bringing with him a cut glass salad bowl. As he handed it over he said, 'I always did think yours was the most difficult course to teach.' I gave the bowl to the parish bazaar.

The summer was over.

2

Autumn

AUTUMN HAS ALWAYS BEEN for me a time of new beginnings. In September I had my hair cut for the first time in six months. I also began to find that I could go for several days without listening to the Beatles – so long as I had Bach (oboe concertos) and Beethoven (cello sonatas). What was hard to take in, however, was that my working life would not start up again as it always did with the end of the summer.

What Mr O. had said about having this happen to me at this point in my life began to make sense. This had hit me not – as often happens – as I was setting out on my adult life, but when I already had a great deal to lose. It seemed a terrible irony that I had taken all these years to achieve a place of safety – only to find that being there made it possible for me to break down. It felt very cruel, and I missed terribly being the person I had become.

'Pain,' I wrote in my journal. 'Just ongoing pain. Keep putting one foot in front of the other.'

It was still difficult for me to get seriously, cleanly angry. As Mr O. had pointed out, other people's feelings always seemed to get in the way of my own: I knew too much about the other people concerned. I was angry with my parents, for example, but they were just as much a mess as I was, so what could they have done about it?

The attack by Perks came, as far as I could see, completely out of the blue: it was simply pain and terror. How could he have dared to attack his own employer's daughter in this way if I had not already been a safe target? It happened after my mother's miscarriage, when she was in the depths of depression and Pete's hair was falling out. Perks must have perceived some level of neglect and thought he could get away with it. Or was he angry with my father about something and punishing me for it?

The seven year old inside me still seemed to want to say something. It was not at all clear what might this be, but at least I knew what had happened to me when I was four. Just as I had comforted my three year old self during the therapy with Patricia, I now spent time sitting and talking with my four year old self. After all, I seemed to be a good enough mother and had been a good enough therapist, and I knew what four year old children were like because I had had one of my own.

By now I had identified three milestones in my story that could be described as abuse: the attack by Perks when I was four; the attempt by Fred, the lodger, to put his hand down my trousers when I was seventeen; and the affair with Corinna which began that Christmas. I now remembered something about the hospital visit when I was fifteen.

It was years since I had even thought about the hospital where I was told I had duodenal ulcers. What I now remembered was lying on my front on a table and two nurses trying to get me lie still: every time they touched my back to try and get me into some sort of position for the examination, I went into a convulsion. They seemed to find this odd and a bit worrying.

Then there was a male doctor and another nurse. There was a hand inside me, pain, and, again, a sense of the nurse being worried. Later, in the kitchen at home, everyone stood around and looked at the purple bruises on my lower abdomen. The whole episode seemed so bizarre that I rang Pete. 'Do you remember when I had to go to the hospital about the duodenal ulcers?' I asked him.

'Yeah, I do. That was a bit weird.'

'Is it true that I had a bruise afterwards?'

'Yes. I remember it vividly. There were purple streaks coming up your abdomen in the shape of a man's hand. It was very strange. No-one knew what to make of it.'

After thinking some more I rang Pete again, this time to ask about Fred, the lodger. What was bothering me was the way I had waited for him to be asked to leave, and yet nothing happened, even after Pete had been sent to talk to him.

'What did happen?' I asked Pete.

'Well, I did go and see him and he didn't deny it. Then he came down to see Deidre and Hugh. I think you must have been out or upstairs. Anyway, they sat round the kitchen table and shared a bottle of whisky with him, and by the time the bottle was empty they had agreed with him that you had been provocative.'

Even now I did not really know how to react. The best I could do was, 'I do think they could have asked me.'

I knew, of course, how common this kind of reaction was with parents of that generation: anything to prevent rocking the boat. But it did hurt, horribly.

Then, of course, there was Corinna. I knew rationally that

what she had done was an abuse of her position, and it had plunged me into a hell from which it took years to recover. Yet it still felt like a kind of redemption. If it had not been for her, I thought, I might never have joined the human race – but how was I to tell? It was not so much the sex that bothered me, but that someone twice my age who knew that she did not love me had taken my all-consuming, passionate, body-heart-and-soul love and treated it as if it were trash. I was aware now of how I had passed some of that hurt on to boyfriends at university – being loved was something I simply could not cope with. Was it that that had made me so convinced I was passing on hurt to the clients in my practice by – as I saw it – abandoning them?

I kept trying to work out what I should be thinking and feeling. That summer the *News of the World* had started naming and shaming sex offenders, which led to riots in Paulsgrove, near Portsmouth, and there had been attacks on people who had abused children. In a small way I was part of that story. I did not know how, knowing what I now knew, I would have reacted if I had been a neighbour of someone who was named. I could not imagine myself living with equanimity close to a known child abuser. Yet the cycle of violence answered by violence depressed me.

What did my religious faith offer me as alternatives to violence? When I had worked with Christian survivors of abuse, 'leaving the judgement to God' seemed a large part of how they not only coped, but also somehow released themselves from a role as victim. In their various ways they had described letting go in the understanding that the judgement belonged to God. What they said had impressed me at the time, though I never fully understood it. Now I decided to ask Richard about it.

Throughout the summer, Richard had continued to be a reliable support. I knew that both he and Mr O. had their boundaries completely in place and that neither of them would ever so much as think of abusing their position: that in itself was one of the most healing things during those months. I needed them both, but it was also quite clear that they had different roles. Although there had been a clear transference of feelings about my father to Richard, and he was an accepting and compassionate listener, it was Mr O. who was my therapist. Now I began to put Richard through his paces as a priest.

Richard was used to me questioning the meaning of everything we said in church. I now began with the 'Our Father', the prayer Nana and my mother had been asking the little girl about in my dream the previous year. Settled in the usual chair in Richard's study, I launched in.

'Every time we say the "Our Father" we say "forgive us our trespasses as we forgive those who trespass against us". What does this mean in this situation? All I can feel is that I have been trespassed against.'

'It does seem to me,' replied Richard slowly, 'that you can't forgive someone who doesn't ask for forgiveness – at least you can't forgive them in such a way as to restore the relationship. Even God can't do that, which is why people confess their sins.'

With Perks, though, surely there was no relationship to be restored. I did not think I could be said to have had a relationship with him before it happened, except that I liked to follow him around and help with the chores in the church. In any case no-one was going to be making any apologies to me. 'So what *can* you do?' I asked. 'Especially

186

when everyone concerned is dead.'

When on tricky ground, Richard was very good at using the word 'we' so that what he said applied to him and everyone else, not just to me. 'I suppose,' he replied, 'we can work on creating a readiness to forgive should the opportunity occur – though that they may never happen, of course.'

'But how do you do that?'

'I think it is about seeing that everyone is a child of God, capable in theory of receiving the light, even if in practice they are cut off from it. By the time we get there, we will have seen something of the light and salvation that is available to us – in spite of, or maybe even because of – what has happened.'

I did not say anything – that 'even because of' was bothering me – and he added, rather dreamily, 'I sometimes wonder if there is a way in which we need to bring forgiveness nearer and nearer to the point where the pain or hurt occurred so that at last it takes place almost during the event.'

Noticing my silence, he smiled and sat up. 'That all sounds very high flown,' he said briskly. Then, in a strange echo of what Mr O. had said about my family he went on, 'I think what it amounts to is that we can only find that place if we know in our hearts that God can make a silk purse out of a sow's ear, and that is all he ever wants to do. So there is nothing wrong with being a sow's ear. It's just the first stage on the way to being something better.'

I came away from this conversation much more upset than I let on. Underneath all his compassion did Richard think that really I was a sow's ear? All the same, it seemed interesting that it might not be necessary to understand at a human level what had happened – I had struggled so hard to do that – but to be able somehow to see the other person in relation to God. Perhaps this was another way of saying what my clients had said about their abusers: I began to understand a little better what they meant.

Psalm 51 came back to me: 'Against Thee [God] only have I sinned.' Could I take it, then, that what had been done to me was not my personal property – it was a crime against God? And did *that* mean that in some fundamental way what Perks did was none of my business? Was this a way of acknowledging the wrong that Perks had done – rather than trying to understand it or explain it away – without harbouring the anger for ever? Thinking this helped me feel a bit less scared of how angry I really was. It is not enough to be a victim, I had discovered: you have to be strong with it.

Yet to think of what Perks had done as like a tile falling off a roof seemed somehow inadequate. Even if it happened within God's Providence and the judgement belonged to God, it was still an act done against me by another human being. In that attack he was my enemy, so what did it mean then to 'Pray for your enemies', as Christ said we should do? I needed a model that could include my anger, at least for the time being.

The next time I saw Richard, I took the discussion a bit further. 'Are you saying that it may not be necessary to understand in a human way how or why someone did something, but only pay attention to the fact that they are made in the image of God and God loves them, and what happens between them and God is none of our business?'

'Something like that, I suppose.'

188

'So the injury is not the personal property of the victim? If you can understand "Against thee [God] only have I sinned" as applying to the person that hurt you, you can acknowledge that what happened was sinful, rather than trying to explain it away?'

'Yes. No-one's saying it wasn't a *sin*.'

'No-one,' Richard had said, 'is saying it wasn't a sin.' Except, perhaps, my father.

After I got home, I talked with my father inside my head and found that it was just fine to feel angry with him on behalf of my four year old self. I told him that it was wrong that she should have had to swallow all the pain and distress of the attack, and experience his disgust. Dealing with all that hurt and anxiety was not my job, but nobody else was doing theirs. It was not me who should have been having panic attacks about violating the sanctuary when I starting going to church again as an adult. I began to be less afraid of my own anger, and found myself rejecting any nonsense about provocation or collusion, whether it was Perks, or Fred or Corinna.

At the same time, Richard's forgiveness model had begun to annoy me. Of course, he had made no demand – or even suggestion – that I should forgive anyone: he had only responded to my questions. Yet I began to feel furious for him for having such grand ideas. Had he ever really forgiven anyone?

That stuff about seeing the light in spite of or maybe because of the pain, and bringing them so close together you forgive even as it is happening. That was a great theory, should you happen to be Christ, but it was asking a hell of a lot of any ordinary person who had been wronged – me in particular. How could it make any sense that I should have forgiven Perks at the moment of the rape? Even now, nearly half a century later, I was going through all the effects of what he had done to me, and there was no way I could simultaneously see Perks as a child of God, just temporarily cut off from light and salvation.

It was obvious even to me that on some level I was angry with Richard simply for being a man, even though I knew he was doing his best. There was, as he himself remarked one day, an awful lot of me very close to the surface. That week I had read an article about husbands beating their wives and using the phrase from Genesis, 'bone of my bone and flesh of my flesh' as a justification for it – using it to mean 'your body is mine to do what I like with'. Why should anyone have to forgive that? So I told Richard about the 'bone of my bone, flesh of my flesh' men.

'I suppose,' he remarked, 'you could say these people are on to something.' Seeing the expression on my face, he added hastily, 'What I mean is they convict themselves, because it says in the Bible, "No man hates his own flesh." To hate your own flesh is a sin.'

'Not so much of a sin as hating someone else's and claiming rights over it, surely?'

Richard grinned. 'You will have to forgive me for speaking theologically,' he said.

'OK', I conceded. '*Theologically*, I think we are agreed that sin is sin, and forgiveness involves acknowledging the damage and letting it go. So you have to feel the anger and all that alongside compassion and love, which can be quite objective things. So that means, does it, that you can accept they are your enemy, and still pray for them because they don't really know what is going on? Is that getting as close as possible to the Christ-on-the-cross position: "Father, forgive, for they know not what they do"?'

Richard was always cautious when it came to identifying too closely with Christ, but he admitted that compassion and love could be objective, and that the Christ-on-the-cross position might be an ideal to arrive at in some far distant future. But I was desperate to be making some sense of all this here and now. At least, I thought, I was doing better than my parents had done. I was undoing some of the denial. Perhaps I deserved some credit for that.

'Meanwhile,' I asked, 'since I find myself going through all this anger, terror and pain is there anything I can do with it? Could you say that letting myself experience that instead of denying it is an on-going act of forgiveness?'

He was not altogether prepared to concede that this was a substitute for what we had been talking about. Although it was annoying that he held back from giving me that satisfaction, one of the things I liked about Richard was that he knew how to stick to his guns.

'Well,' he said, 'I think we have to bear in mind how important it is to restore the image of God that Adam and Eve saw in each other before the Fall. It was that that made it possible for the devil to tempt them – and then of course that vision was lost, along with so many other things. Part of our return to where we should be is recovering that ability to see the image of God in other people.'

'But what if they are hiding it so that you can't see it?'

'It's a problem,' he admitted. 'You have to remember that for us forgiveness is always going to be either incomplete or temporary. You always have to return to it and renew it.'

'That does sound a bit depressing.' I could see this

stretching out for the rest of my life. Always having to return and renew my bloody forgiveness. Did Richard really understand, I wondered, what was going on for me? – or was I making something out of nothing, just making a big fuss about things that people just have to live with all the time? I began to sink into despair.

Richard must have sensed something because he changed gear. 'I'll try and say a bit more,' he began, and leaned forward in his chair. 'All I've got that I can relate to what you seem to be struggling with is that all through my teens I lived in a kind of blind rage towards my father. I was utterly mad.'

Richard? Who was always so calm and transparent? He went on, 'He hasn't changed at all, but I have made peace with him. He is what he always was – a quiet, inward man, perhaps a bit disappointed in me because he doesn't understand where I have ended up.

'With my mother, though, it's different. She was not much help to us, and I threatened to kill her once – by post. I can't say that I have more than partially forgiven her even after all these years. But I am in better shape now than I was even twenty years ago. Things do move on, even late in the game.' He stopped abruptly and sat back. 'I'm not sure I can say anything else.'

It was, however, a great deal. Threatened to kill his mother, did he? By *post*? I knew nothing about his family history, but however different his experience might be, he had definitely joined me on my side of the fence.

3

Paddy

WHATEVER THEOLOGY MIGHT SAY, my psyche was still far from satisfied. Mr O. came back from his holiday, and with the resumption of our sessions came fresh surges of anger and fear. The dreams also kept coming thick and fast, three or four a night:

> *Two families: one is Mafioso, the other their victims. The revenge of the Mafia family is closing in. All is fear, tension, violence in the air. What is going to be done to whom? I am particularly terrified for my sister who is sexually inexperienced. What will they do to her?*
>
> *There is a room with several of the Mafia men on the bed, and my sister is sent into it. At first I am relieved they don't seem to be going to do anything to her. Then she is grabbed by a 'bestial' brother in a lower bunk bed .....*

When I woke from this dream my back was in spasm and I was full of wind.

That day I had a cranial osteopathy session. The way I thought of it was that apart from Jim, who was keeping a roof over my head, there were three people caring for me: Mr O. was caring for my mind, Lydia for my body, and Richard for my spirit. Of the three, the cranial work was the least painful. I lay on a couch, fully clothed, while Lydia placed her hands wherever she sensed they were needed, asking an occasional question as a result of what she encountered but otherwise uninterested in my story: she left the inside of my head free and I liked that. Nevertheless, whatever she did, mysterious though it was, sometimes produced powerful sensations.

The morning after the Mafioso dream Lydia remarked that it was hard to get a flow of energy between my top half and my bottom half. These blockages could occur, she explained, when there has been damage in the past that leads to a build-up of tension in the tissues. Would I be willing to try working with two therapists, one at each end of me, to see if a connection could be made?

I agreed, and at the next session, she introduced her colleague, Gabriella. When I lay on the couch, Lydia sat behind me and placed her hands around my head, while Gabriella slid hers under my pelvis. Before long Gabriella asked, 'Have you ever been in a high velocity car crash?'

The answer was no, and we continued in silence, the two women at either end of me gently working on the flows of energy between the two halves of my body while I stared at the ceiling. After a few minutes, tears began to pour from my eyes, and first Lydia and then Gabriella also began to weep copiously. While this was going on a name rose up from my pelvis into my brain: Paddy. My mother's brother. My policeman uncle.

As Pete had said, 'Paddy was cheery like Herman Goering, that jolly old Nazi.' He was different from the rest of the family: neither religious nor depressed, and his aggression was all on the surface. After Nana died, he and my mother had an argument over the price of the coffin (she wanted the most expensive, he the cheapest) and did not speak to each other for seventeen years. 'He was such as nice boy', my mother used to say, 'until he started doing that milk round and got in with that milkman'.

Yet something in me had a kind of affinity with Paddy. It was not that I did not think he was as bad as everyone else did. It was more that the others seemed to wonder why he was such an angry person while it seemed obvious to me, given the poverty and pain he had grown up with. When his name floated up from my gut, I could not help wondering if he was the missing link in the seven year old story. So what was going on when I was seven?

Around that time, Paddy was going through a bitter divorce, and was often in and out of our house. His girlfriend, Frankie, was a bottle blonde who clanked with costume jewellery wherever she went. My mother told me that Frankie was so jealous of Paddy's daughter, Sadie, that she used to hide her jewellery and accuse Sadie of stealing it. Paddy would then beat Sadie as a punishment.

One day it was announced that Frankie was going to have an operation for a bad back.

'What are they going to do?' someone asked, and Paddy replied, 'They will lay her on her front on a bed at the end of the ward, and they'll draw a target on her back. Then all the doctors will line up at the other end of the ward with a javelin, and they'll run the length of the ward and try to get the javelin into the bullseye.'

Night after night I lay awake in terror, thinking about what he had said. Whatever happened, I must make sure I never had to go to hospital. Did everyone eventually have to go to hospital? Nana had. My mother had. My father never had as far as I knew. I went over and over in my mind the grown-ups I knew, working out who had managed to stay out of hospital and who hadn't. I never said a word to anyone about what was keeping me awake. It was only clear that I could not get to sleep.

My mother tried to help by winding up my musical box that played 'Annie Laurie'. I had longed for this musical box: when you opened it there was a little mirror in the lid, and a plastic ballet dancer who rotated while the music played. Before long, though, I could not bear to hear it: it had become associated with my terror about Frankie's operation and just filled me with dread.

Did Paddy come up to my room one night – or several? 'I'll give you something to help you sleep ...'? I had no memory. I just felt intensely aware of him, and he felt somehow close, as though he had put something really bad inside me. Even now I needed the bedroom door to stay open so I would hear if anyone was coming up the stairs.

Once more Pete was the person to ask. Did he think there was any possibility that there might have been some kind of abuse (of me by Paddy)? He laughed grimly. 'Yes,' he said, 'not impossible at all.'

I told him about the session with Lydia and Gabriella. 'Well, yeah,' he said, in an unsurprised tone. He told me about when Deidre last saw Paddy after she and Paddy had started speaking again. He and Frankie were still together – if you could call it that. He sat in a large chair from which he could barely move because he was now so obese, swilling Special Brew and clicking the TV remote. Frankie was thin as thin, scuttling about with her now scraggy hair still dyed blonde, and her bracelets still clanking. She was terrified of Paddy and kept a bottle of gin in the kitchen cupboard, regularly slipping off to take a swig. Deidre arrived with a quart of whisky in her handbag and there was some competition, Pete said, for who could get the kitchen to themselves for a secret tipple. The food was mountainous, and Deidre was unable to eat it. Too scared to say anything she shovelled quantities of it into her handbag. It was not long after this that Paddy died of a heart attack, and that was all I was ever to know about his later life.

For the first time in months, meanwhile, the inside of my mouth began to relax. There were whole chunks of time when I was not plagued by *globus hystericus*, and this was an indescribable relief. The back pain, however, continued to get worse in spite of the cranial work, where there was a lot of movement inside me, and a sense of my top half and bottom half beginning to join up. That is, the pain now ran right through me. It was, I imagined, rather like what it would be like when sensation begins to return to someone who has been paralysed by nerve damage. Nevertheless, I continued to have a lot of lower back pain, as though something inside me was locked in an uncomfortable position, so I mentioned this to Lydia.

'Yes,' said she said, 'I can feel it. It is like a deep body memory of the body recoiling in horror'.

That weekend, I spent a night at a friend's house in London and had a dream which seemed to tell the story of my life:

A young woman, blonde, slim, attractive. She is having to consult a doctor, and has seen a series of doctors before she comes to this one avuncular consultant. He says she may have to have an internal examination. She confides in him that she is terrified and he is reassuring. Then he goes ahead and does the examination in a violent, sexy way. She is confused and kisses him. He walks out in disgust.

Was it possible that this was an echo of what happened with my uncle Paddy?

Before I caught the train home I went on impulse into a church where confessions were being heard in old fashioned confessionals, like the ones I had known as a child. I went into one of the little cubicles with a priest behind the grille, and knelt down. He said the opening prayers, but I was then unable to speak and simply wept.

'What is it,' he asked eventually.

'I was raped as a child,' I managed to say, and spilled out some story about my uncle abusing me and my parents doing nothing about it, knowing as I said it that I did not know if it was even true. I needed to say it anyway. The priest's response was instantaneous.

'You do not have to be the scapegoat of this terrible family,' he told me. 'Do not be afraid of your anger. I am your witness, even at the Day of Judgement that you have not sinned in this.'

It was a dramatic but heartening response from a stranger, and I was moved by it, and by receiving absolution. It was a pity, then, that when I left the confessional he followed me out from his side, took my hand and asked if I would like to talk further. I have no doubt that he meant well, but what I needed from him just then was to remain a stranger.

Part 6
SHIFTING

1

Spasm

As AUTUMN SLID INTO WINTER I was coming to realise that this was not simple burn out: I could not just recover from it and get on with my life. I would never again be the person I was a year before. It was very frightening.

Since there was no question of going back to practising as a therapist, I began to take in admin and editorial work from some of Jim's customers. The pay was minimal, but I could do it at home in my own time and it did not involve having to relate to other people. Having some work also helped me feel less contaminated: there was still something I could contribute that people valued

My body was far from well, however. The muscle spasms continued and I often needed to lie on the floor to get comfortable. Sometimes I had to walk with a stick.

'I think,' said Lydia, 'that the spasm is your body protecting you from feelings that are unmanageable.'

Unconvinced, I went again to see Dr Gibson, who reluctantly suggested that Valium might relieve the muscle spasm. I still struggled to take Prozac, and after Pete's experience Valium was even more frightening, but I was desperate for anything that would help the pain, and took the prescription to the pharmacy. Later that morning when a therapist friend called round for coffee, I mentioned my misgivings. 'But it's lovely stuff,' he told me. 'Let's see what size pills they've given you.'

I showed him the bottle and he laughed. 'You don't want to worry about those,' he said. 'You could safely take those in handfuls.'

Pete's attitude was less relaxed. 'It is such dreadful stuff when it gets hold of you. I've got a friend who is trying to come off it. She gets so desperate she shaves bits off a pill with a razor blade and takes those, just to get something inside her.'

I remained cautious but I did use it from time to time. It gave me a few hours now and then of dreamless sleep, and enabled me to sit down comfortably for short periods.

Something new had started to happen in my dreams in amongst the seemingly endless nightmares. About every two weeks I found myself looking at a place of indescribable beauty: a river or hillside, the edge of the sea or a forest. It was different each time, but every time it was in some sense my own, and to see it filled me with delight. Although it was always at a distance or something stopped me reaching it, its very existence gave me hope.

In waking life it helped that both Lydia and Mr O. were using the words 'sexual abuse'. I still found it hard to believe I was, as it were, entitled to them.

In a session with Mr O. towards the end of September, I went through the whole story of Corinna in one go, and suddenly felt – for the first time – really angry about what she had done. I was – as Mr O. had remarked years before – 'boiling with rage,' but this was a new rage I never even knew was there. What Corinna did, I thought to myself, was terrible. I was seventeen, and grieving for my grandmother who had been like a mother to me, and I needed someone to talk to, not sex. I had even said to someone once – not in anger, but humorously – 'Maybe she had sex with me to shut me up about death'. Talking with Mr O. that day it occurred to me for the first time that she *could have just listened*.

It was also a new thought that I might have been in need of comfort. My mother was so devastated by Nana's death that she had no sympathy to spare. When I came out in a rash after the funeral she asked why I had it and I replied that I thought it might be stress. She looked at me with incomprehension and asked, 'What have you got to be stressed about?'

The next time I saw Richard I told him about being suddenly angry with Corinna and that it seemed to me this was the first time I had said no to colluding with what was done to me. This seemed to cheer him up enormously.

'You are absolutely right,' he said, 'There can be no collusion! All collusion is with distortion, fallenness, and it's basically a dead end.' He went on to say something which at last affirmed the idea that coming through this might be in itself a form of forgiveness. 'It will be a marvellous thing,' he said, 'to have lived through all this and not just survived but to have made a real life of it.'

Lying on the floor while my muscles slowly released the spasm I found myself talking to my body, telling it that at last it could let this stuff go. *You don't have to hold on to these terrible secrets any more. They have been told, and no-one has rejected me or disbelieved me or blamed me. Indeed no-one has murdered me.* These were amazing and heartening facts.

I wrapped up Corinna's chess set which she had left with me before she emigrated in 1971, and gave it to the parish bazaar, that repository of all unmanageable objects. All my adult life I had felt the pain of Corinna not loving me. Now it seemed I could let her be, as someone who did not love me – but I did not want the possessions of someone who did not love me occupying my space.

Then, one evening, a violent attack of sneezing seemed to clear the remaining back spasm. The nightmares began to recede, and sleep to return. A dream also suggested something was shifting:

> *I have gone to stay in a large house, which is partly St George's vicarage. It is run by two sisters: one dark, powerful and mad, and the other shadowy and subservient. A lot of people go off to Paddy's funeral. I decide I am not well enough and stay behind with the two sisters. We prepare food for the funeral meal and people come back and eat it. There is a lot left over.*

> *I decide to go for a walk, and downstairs the dark sister is with a little girl. She says sharply to the little girl, 'Come here!' The girl does not move and she says it more sharply. I know this is wrong, but I smile at the little girl in an encouraging sort of way (just as my mother used to do in difficult situations) and she goes to the sister who grabs her and slaps her hard.*

> *I feel despairing and guilty because I have colluded. I decide to leave, and later I am driving away. There does not seem to be anything I can do.*

In the dream, Paddy was dead. He was no longer living

inside me, and I could even allow myself not to be well enough to go to the funeral. There was a lot of funeral food left over, however – or you could say it was undigested.

As for the two sisters, their presence suggested that two aspects of me were differentiating. In some ways it was a classic victim – persecutor – rescuer dream. The rescuer – myself/the shadowy sister – was ineffective against the persecutor of the little girl. There was that moment when I smiled. I could see my mother smiling like that: as Pete had said, *No word of correction if you were being naughty while you were out: just this terrible unexpected* Stuka *attack on the way home.* It was Pete's memory, but the same mother. The great thing about the dream as far as I was concerned was that I accepted there was nothing I could do, and left.

In waking life, too, I was getting over the feeling that I was a total pariah for whom nothing was bad enough, though I was still oscillating between anger and contrition towards my father. It felt as though a voice on a weak wavelength was trying to get through to tell me that his ultimate verdict was that he loved me. In a ritual act that briefly provided some relief, I went and cleared my parents' grave, and planted some flowers there.

By now I reckoned that I was not clinically depressed, and went to see Dr Gibson again to talk about stopping the Prozac. She agreed I was much better than I had been, but said I had to be well for six months before coming off it. However, I could reduce the dose so long as I monitored my symptoms and saw her once a month. This was both reassuring and alarming. *I really had been ill, then.* The remaining Valium I took back to the pharmacy, much to Pete's relief.

The signs of recovery were noticed by my friend and colleague Toby, and he tried to persuade me to take part in teaching a sexuality course in January: 'You'll be ready by then,' he assured me.

'But I don't want to have to be ready.'

'You could do it now if you had to. You'll have me to look after you, and you can do as much or as little as you like.'

I was touched by his request and promised to think about it. Even more, however, I was pleased with myself that I did not need to say yes just yet. My friends and colleagues wanted me back. I wanted that myself: although still fragile, I was getting bored with this story, and with the past. But I did not want to take 'a flight into health'. I had gone too far into sickness to settle for anything short of true recovery. When I asked Richard what he thought about taking part in the course, he shared my caution.

'You know,' he said, 'that I am fairly primitive in my views on the human psyche, but it does seem to me you have plenty to get on with. Why not relax and deal with what is already in hand? I do believe God provides the material we need to move on if we are just attentive enough.'

I told Toby that I would not be working on the course this year, at least. I was still doing what Andrew had called my 'other job'.

By December, I could look back and see just how ill I had been. As far as Perks was concerned, alongside a new sense of outrage that this should have happened to me (an achievement in itself), I was deeply angry that these things were still happening to children now. I was beginning to understand in a new way what it meant to be a child, and what was lost for me in that attack and its aftermath. I was also beginning to smoke less. Cigarettes had been vital in containing my feelings: now they seemed less necessary, and some days I did not smoke at all.

The seven year old story was still – and would remain – a mystery apart from my suspicions about Paddy. And although nightmares were still presenting violent images or short pieces of narrative: they were more objective than before. The violence happened at more of a distance.

For the first time since I became ill I went away alone, to a retreat house in Somerset where I had been before. Half way there I had a major panic attack and had to stop at a friend's house for the night. But I did make it to Somerset, where I did a lot of staring into space while the rain poured down outside my window. By the time I got back home it seemed to me that I was fed up with talking about myself, and having my body explored by Lydia. I wanted to go inside myself and sort things out there. I brought the cranial work and the sessions with Mr O. to an end.

Mr O. was clearly concerned, but had no choice but to accept that all I wanted right then was to leave the whole story behind as far as possible.

'Remember,' he said to me in our last session, 'you are trying to divest yourself of these people.' This made an impression, but it was only years later that I really began to understand how important that was.

Given my tendency to separation anxiety my constant desire to shed Mr O. was interesting. He was, of course, extremely important, though I did not allow myself to acknowledge it. I kept coming closer, breaking off, and going back again in a way that was quite different from my anxious attachment to Patricia. This was a classic case of avoidant attachment. He was certainly very secure for me, and I did not expect him to disappear when I was away from him. I knew he would be there for me when I wanted him. I was also grateful to him. At the same time, I needed to keep him at a distance. Was there some deep distrust because I knew he had been a priest? Yet I trusted Richard implicitly and he was a priest. Whatever was going on, I insisted on stopping the therapy. And I was not happy when Richard, too, thought this might be premature. Eager to explain to him that I was right, I even wrote him a letter to ram the point home:

When I woke up this morning, after a good, deep sleep, I felt safe and located in my life and in my home in a way that I have never felt in waking life before ...
I know enough about the facts of what was done to me. The remaining 'issue' is my relationship with my father and how it was lost and how I got lost in the process. Now I can look at my parents and family history in a new way .....

Of course I have been asking myself whether I am avoiding or acting out a transference with Mr O. but I honestly don't think so. I told you that when we started work in March I talked to him about how cross I had been with him for saying I was a 'going concern' twelve years before. He was very good with it and encouraged me through the process of breakdown, giving me permission not to be a going concern.

Yet what I felt when I realised I was not going to see him this morning is that I am a going concern, and that is all right because it's different. I don't have to keep the world from falling apart. It did that last year, and not only have I survived but many things have improved ...

Of course I don't mean that I have suddenly become well overnight, but I do believe I am ready to go forwards not backwards ....

Richard did not respond.

The approach of Christmas brought memories of the visits to my mother and clearing her house – the same memories that had haunted my fall into depression the year before – and I struggled not to sink emotionally. Hanging on to what Mr O. had said, I wrote on a piece of paper: 'Divest yourself of the past; move through the present into the future' and kept it in my room. Kathy and her boyfriend were making Christmas arrangements for both families: when I watched them at work, all my sadness and anxiety melted away. This was the present. The other stuff was the past.

2

Full Fathom Five thy Father Lies

EARLY IN THE NEW YEAR Pete and I went out for lunch and had a long conversation about our father. Over Christmas I had been in touch with a priest who had worked with Hugh as a curate, and asked him what that was like. It was fine, he said, as long as you fitted in with Hugh's world view: 'He had decided how the world is, and if you did not fit in with that you did not exist.'

As an example, he told me a story of a neighbouring priest who had been dying of AIDS. When it was suggested to my father, who was then Rural Dean, that this man might need counselling, he rejected it straight off, saying, 'He has been to confession, and that is enough.'

This description stirred something in me, and I wanted to know how Pete reacted to it. 'Yes,' he said, 'that is very accurate. His feelings were kept very deep down. There was one time, though' he went on, 'when I remember being aware of his feelings. It was in the early 80s, when he was quite depressed. There was a lot in the news about an eleven year old girl who was raped and murdered on her way home from a riding lesson. It preyed on Hugh's mind, and rocked his faith.'

This was fascinating. Did it mean that somewhere

deep down my father did know about me being raped by Perks and his own lack of reaction? Did the way this story affected him mean he really did love me? It also made me angry. Why did Pete know all this, and Hugh never shared any of it with me?

We went on to talk about our grandfather. 'I have wondered,' I said, 'whether there was any funny business with Auntie Cordelia – incest I mean with Grandpa. All that 'can't keep a maid' business and Cordelia never allowed to leave home until they had both died.'

'It's not impossible' replied Pete, as he had done when I asked him about Paddy.

'Do you remember,' I went on, 'how when she came to stay after he died, she was always groping us. If you sat on the sofa next to her she would reach out and stroke us – not in a normal way – it was really vigorous. It was quite scary. As though she did not even know she was doing it.'

'Yeah, I do remember that. It was kind of weird.'

'Grandpa wasn't much of a role model to Hugh for being a father.'

'Hugh really hated him,' Pete said. 'Remember when Cordelia brought his ashes up to us to be buried? We drove to the cemetery. And Hugh opened the boot of the car, grabbed a box and threw it at me. He said, "Here's your grandfather – catch." I did catch it, thank God. He was such a strange guy. Part of it must have been all that public school stuff. He was like people who come back from the war and are totally in denial about what has gone on.'

Pete and I had buried Cordelia's ashes in a family grave with those of her parents, as she had requested in her will. Suddenly I wanted to go and get them and bury them nearer my home, away from them. 'Do you remember

Hugh ever really expressing his feelings?' I asked.

'Yeah, there was one time. It was during the miners' strike, when Mrs T. brought in Ian MacGregor to deal with them, and I asked him what he felt about that, and he said "It is inappropriate."'

I waited for the rest of the story, but that was it.

'That was your one memory of your father expressing his feelings?' I asked in a mock shocked tone worthy of Mr O. Pete shifted on his chair.

'Well, it was the way he said it.'

We ate some pizza in silence. Then Pete put down his knife and fork. 'Did you know,' he asked, 'that our grandfather ran a prison camp for German soldiers during World War I?'

'No.' How did he know all this stuff and I didn't? 'And I never did understand why Hugh wasn't in the army. Deirdre always said it was because he was training as a priest.'

'I don't know,' said Pete. 'I heard somewhere that he was rejected for military service because of grossness and obesity, and that he was supposed to be diabetic.'

'Diabetic?' I thought of the large and infrequent meals we consumed in the vicarage, the twice a day alcohol. 'But he couldn't have been diabetic and lived as he did – he'd have been in a coma.'

Pete shrugged. 'God knows what it actually was, but I hated it that he wasn't in the war. In all my friends' houses there was always some misty-eyed hero who had been in the army or air force or whatever. But not Hugh. He was a bloody air raid warden. Spent the war knitting dishcloths in f-ing air raid shelters.'

We talked some more about Hugh's parents. Our grandmother, anorectic, sexless, pious, grooming Hugh for the priesthood, and our grandfather who resented this. He was always vicious to Hugh about his lack of money. There were stories – told by Deidre – of our parents struggling to make ends meet, and of her persuading Hugh to ask his father for help, and his father telling him to get a proper job if he wanted to earn a decent wage.

'Muck to brass to muck in three generations,' said Pete. 'Deidre used to go on about them sleeping in twin beds – our parents never did that.'

'But she and Hugh always had a bolster between them, 'I said. 'She said that it was because Hugh lashed out in his sleep. Do you remember those mysterious bruises she used to have on her upper arms?'

'He didn't know his own strength,' replied Pete. 'Do you remember that "horse bite" business?'

I had forgotten, but now it came back. How Hugh would grab your thigh just above the knee and squeeze very hard on a nerve until he could see it was really hurting. Then he would laugh and say 'Horse bite'.

'Of course,' Pete went on, 'there was also that time he was supposed to have thyroid trouble and Deidre made him come off the pills because they turned him into a violent sexual monster.'

'When was that?' I had never heard about it before. It felt as though Pete had been alive during our childhood and I had been locked in some kind of bubble.

'Oh, sometime in the fifties.' After a pause, he added, 'We've never really talked about him before, have we.'

'No.'

'But he was the safe one. We needed to keep him safe. He was always the sane one, the reliable one, yet he was in quite a mess really. '

After this conversation, I went back to a book about incest, and it mapped the whole emotional landscape of my life. I could sign up to all the indications – the nightmares, fear of basements, hypervigilance – but didn't everyone have those in some degree? Something had happened that mixed up sex and pain in my head as things a man does to a woman: something, I was sure, in those Latin lessons in Hugh's study, which began when I was seven. I was excited by Latin grammar and worked hard. After that, there was a fleeting something about not knowing something I should know about Roman history. *They turned him into a violent sexual monster – I don't know – sometime in the fifties …* If there was a man who was a seething volcano of sexual frustration and an adoring over-sexualised daughter, perhaps anything was possible. Most likely it was a physical attack – some kind of punishment – rather than actual incest, but as with Paddy, I would never actually know.

Even I realised I needed to go back to Mr O., but I waited a week or two because I was simply too angry to contemplate sitting in a room and talking with him about it. I was not consciously angry with him: I respected and trusted him – but at the same time I had a feeling that any therapy was simply going to shut me up, prevent me from telling the truth. I also felt waves of rage against Patricia. She had been wonderful at the mother transference, but she had never seemed to want to know about my father. Everyone, it seemed, was protecting him and silencing me.

Aileen's words kept coming back to me, 'You have been horribly betrayed' and another psalm verse kept running in my mind: 'If it had been an enemy that had done this, then I could have borne it, but it was thou, my own

212

familiar friend. We kept sweet counsel together and walked in the house of God as friends'. That was just it. Perks was an enemy and essentially didn't matter. But Hugh and I loved the church together, even before I started playing the organ. Every Good Friday when I was still young, we walked together in the vicarage garden and talked about what the day meant. And every Holy Week he would get all the parish children – me included – to act out the Passion story in the chancel and side chapel of the church. He was very good at this, and I loved it. He was also good at making up stories. There was a whole other family he made up who had great adventures, and when he had time or if I was ill he would come and sit on the bed and tell me about them.

Nevertheless, when I tried to think about these things they were overlaid by a cold, frozen anger which went back a long way, as though at some point in my childhood I simply removed myself from him.

How I wanted to forget all this stuff! I sickened on thinking about it, and told myself it was self-indulgent. For the first time since all this began, I started to question what I was doing in the Church. The real damage and betrayal had happened in the church and from within the Church. It was true that alongside the treatment I had received, the Church had held me through the experiences of the previous months, not only in the person of Richard but in the community I belonged to and its theology and its liturgy. Without it I could well have needed to be in hospital. Yet why had I walked straight into the lions' den?

I rang Richard and asked if he knew about reaction formation.

'I've heard the phrase,' he admitted, 'but I've never understood what it means.'

'Well, I think what Freud meant by it was that you have a feeling about someone – you are angry, say – and it is so powerful that it scares you. You are afraid of what you might do to them. So you react to the person in the opposite way, and are extra nice to them – except you don't, of course, realise what in fact you are doing.'

'Makes sense to me.'

'I've been wondering, you see, if I kind of fell in love with the Church because of what had happened before, and really I was just terribly angry. Maybe my whole relationship with the Church is reaction formation?'

I longed for him to say no, of course not, but he was too wise for that. 'I simply don't know,' he replied.

One thing that bothered me about the whole religious enterprise was that it seemed geared to spending eternity with God, and this, unfortunately, was an idea filled me with dread. It was true that my experience of sitting with my mother while she was dying, and the glimpses I had had of joy and beauty during the acute phase of my illness could make it all seem worthwhile. Yet I could see ahead of me a lifetime – perhaps an eternity – of struggle to live with and accommodate both good and evil, when I actually simply longed to despair and stop struggling to make sense of it all. Again I found myself wondering about my mother. There were many levels on which she never gave up – in relation to Uncle Jimmy for example, or in her determination to keep her own home – but the despair – the depression, the drugs and the alcohol – won.

It now seemed providential that when I was caring for her I did not know what I now knew, because unless I had already come through it I would not have been able to do what I did. But it left me with a strange sensation of being 'had' – that everyone knew except me what had happened to me. Richard was interested by this idea. 'I suppose,' he remarked, 'that we are all 'had' by God, because we don't actually have a clue what is really going on – we just have to trust that it is for our ultimate benefit.'

It was like being pulled between two poles of a magnet. Sometimes it seemed that all religion was corrupt and only psychotherapy could help me through. At others all my old rage against therapy returned and it seemed that only religion – and liturgy in particular – could save me.

It was February before I could bring myself to make an appointment with Mr O., and immediately the muscle spasms began again, as though my body was panicking at the idea of talking to him.

3

2001 – Back to the Consulting Room

THE NIGHT AFTER I arranged to see Mr O. again, I had a dream that began with a verse from Psalm 5, though it continued rather differently:

> *'My throat is an open sepulchre'. I am reaching down into it and pulling out handfuls of gunge which is filling up my lungs. I have got near the bottom of my lungs now and am worried that reaching inside like this will give me a lung infection (though I think this may be treatable). At the bottom there is more stuff, but I am close to my insides – can I remove it without damaging me? It is utterly disgusting. Towards the end of the dream I am surprised I can get inside my body like this.*

For several days after this dream I once more kept falling into physical shock – cold and shivering. It was different from the shock that had wiped me out the previous year, and felt more like body memory making itself known. For the first time it occurred to me that I might have swallowed Perks' semen. *Why do I feel as though I have inhaled ground glass?*

As well as seeing Mr O. I also went back to the 'double' cranial work. Lydia was a liminal kind of person

216

around whom synchronicities tended to occur. In the middle of my treatment the doorbell rang and she said to Gabriella, 'That's the boiler man.'

For a moment I thought she meant Perks, the 'boiler man' who had threatened to throw me in the flames. When we were coming to the end of the session Lydia remarked that whereas a few months before my head had been like an unexploded bomb, it now felt as though the explosion was happening. This certainly made sense to me.

It also got me interested in the whole idea of recovery. This was a new idea, in the sense that until now I had thought you simply had to enlarge yourself to absorb more and more pain. Now I began to realise that something radically different might be taking place: perhaps my psyche knew what to do to recover, and was getting on with the job almost regardless of me. I was still angry but it had a different quality to it. I could name the things that had happened to me as being bad things. I rejected them, and they were more and more outside me instead of possessing my whole self.

In late February there was a dream in which I met a six year old girl. This was exciting, as before this I had had no access to myself at this age. If I tried to go back there, I turned into a boy. But here she was, my six year old self. In the dream she was asking why I wasn't interested in her. She had no clothes, and she wanted me to know what was going on in the small of her back.

All through the following day I talked to her in my head, comforted her, and helped her to get dressed. The next night I had another dream:

I meet Pete outside St George's vicarage. He is in his

school uniform and is about ten, which makes me six or seven. We go into the house, and there I experience the same kind of attack from behind as happened in my dream last autumn, only this time I am trapped and subjected to something horribly painful. There are some vague healing figures who are looking on and want to help.

This dream was as close as I got, or probably ever will get, to any direct memory of what happened when I was seven. I did not know it was possible to feel such physical pain in a dream, but it was also something familiar, something I had known about and been afraid of all my life. *Fear of breakdown is the fear of something that has already happened.* I was grateful that there were healing figures in the dream, but I nevertheless spent the rest of the night shivering and my muscles were in a bad way in the morning. A week later there was another dream:

There is a man having an affair with a woman. She lives by a river. She is found dead, stabbed in her bed, and there is a murder hunt.

Eventually I am visited by the police and there is an interview in which we sit around a table with my parents. I am charged with the murder. I agree that I did it, and that there was a turning point when I went into the house with a knife.

So, I am the murderer, the perpetrator. My parents sit around a table and accuse me. *They agreed you were provocative.* As Mr O. had said, I did not need anyone to accuse me, the judgement was all there inside me. These dreams brought with them waves of shame and self-disgust: my very right to exist was in doubt. I clung to the idea of the people close to me who knew my story and did

218

not turn away, Mr O., Richard and Toby in particular.

Terrible though they were, the quality of these feelings was different from the previous summer. They were more mature, more differentiated – more like the feelings of a seven year old than a four year old. I had not disappeared into limbo as I did the previous summer: whatever was going on, I was still here. I decided to carry on with Prozac for the time being.

By now I was much less concerned than I had been about understanding forgiveness, recognising perhaps that it was just too difficult, or at least premature. I had come across Psalm 137, 'By the waters of Babylon …' which ends, 'Happy shall he be who requites you with what you have done to us! Happy shall he be who takes your little ones and dashes them against the rock!' This verse upsets people so much that it is often omitted when the psalm is used in church. When it is used, it is often interpreted in spiritual terms: the 'little ones' are sinful thoughts which should be stopped before they became fully formed.

I, however, luxuriated in its anger. *No*, I thought, *this is not some spiritual statement. It is for real. It would have been better if Paddy had never been born. It would have been better if his children had never been born. He was a monster. That is how I feel, and I cannot pretend I feel otherwise. Yes, I am a murderer, but that's how it is. This psalm says: 'I am angry, murderously angry, and I am going to say so.' It says – and I say – to God, 'This is how angry I am, and I can't do better than this. You deal with it.'*

Another thing Winnicott said besides his comment on the fear of breakdown, was that it is important to take hatred as seriously as love. Now with Mr O., I began to think about ways I might have expressed my murderous feelings as a child. I remembered that I used to pass wind frequently and loudly, especially when there were visitors.

'Was that an aeroplane?' a visiting bishop once asked during dinner after one of my spectacular farts. I could visualise the scene, all of us sitting around the table with me opposite him in his purple stock. When I looked for myself in this scene, however, there was no little girl sitting in my place, only a boy in a school blazer. That did not trouble Mr O. He knew it was me. 'Everyone heard,' he remarked, 'But no-one *heard*.'

This was astonishing. He could take seriously a message that I did not even know *was* a message. He really did think I had something to say.

At last there came a night when I managed to scream 'No!' and wake myself up before the pain came instead of going into spasm. I had held on to myself and not given way.

Lying on the floor, I thought again about my father. Yes, as a child I had adored him. As I stayed with that thought, something happened deep inside a muscle in my lower back which I can only describe as an explosion, like a firework going off. Something had been blown open. For days afterwards I was beset by a great, undifferentiated sadness, and a temptation not to exist. It took all my strength to resist that, forcing myself to look at the facts as I knew them.

Whatever actually happened, my father let me down. And though I adored him, I hardly knew him. No-one did: he was encased in loneliness. I wondered if anyone loved him. Perhaps Aunt Cordelia? It was hard to put Deidre and 'love' in the same sentence.

My father's presence could be comforting because it was so solid, but he was often like a thundercloud waiting to burst. I remembered the old Hoover we had when I was a child, with its brown dust bag that swelled up when it was switched on. It petrified me. In my final year at Oxford, when I shared a house with my friend Jane, I lay awake night after night convinced that the immersion heater was going to explode. It was impossible to decide which was more frightening: to risk explosion or to wake Jane, who would certainly be annoyed. Eventually the college doctor gave me Mogadon, pills with tiny little shut eyes sketched on them and I began to laugh myself to sleep. Yes, I had always been terrified of explosions – but so had Hugh. When the IRA bombing campaign began in London he never got in his car without looking underneath it to make sure no-one had planted something there.

In what had been my consulting room was the desk from Hugh's study which I had taken to my house when my mother moved out of the vicarage. Without letting myself stop to think, I called in the auctioneers and arranged for them to take it away for sale. That afternoon I got the two landscape paintings by my mother out of the attic and had a bonfire in the garden of them along with a portrait of my paternal grandfather. *Remember you are trying to divest yourself of these people.*

It was autumn again, a year since the dream which had first sent my muscles into spasm. My rage gave me a sense of affinity with Paddy: you did not just have to get depressed in response to tragedy – you could get angry instead, which was what he did. I could see now, as well, the pain I had passed on to other people after Corinna.

'It's quite easy,' I said to Richard, 'to see how Paddy became an abuser. I am in touch enough with my own self-hatred to see how easily you would pass the hatred on if you can't express it any other way. The secrecy makes us go on falling into it unless something can break through it.'

Richard did not say much but a few days later, at my request, he held a small prayer service for my dead family members.

'I want you to understand,' I said when we made the arrangement, 'that this is both a yes and a no. Yes, we all shared the same inheritance and they are entitled to honour as ancestors. But no, I do not share their way of dealing with the mess we all found ourselves in, and I must free myself of that.'

I took several things with me to the service: my friend from church, Annie, a photo of Paddy and the one of my father dressed as a pantomime dame, a box of matches and a large rocket. After the service we all went out to the church garden where I ripped up the photos and burnt them. Then we let off the rocket.

4

A New Year

BY THE SPRING OF 2002, I was thinking about expanding my editorial work into a separate business alongside Jim's. With careful monitoring from Dr Gibson I had come off Prozac, and was also thinking about working towards an ending with Mr O. The cranial osteopathy had come to an end when the back pain returned around Christmas: Lydia said that this time I needed to get medical help. By February I could hardly walk and my right foot was numb. There were days when I could not sit at all, but I was able to lie on the sofa and use a lap top.

None of this was surprising. I knew from working with other people that when you recover deeply repressed memories of physical abuse, psychological processing may not be enough. Sometimes the body needs its own healing too. After the memories come up there might be bladder trouble, mouth problems or investigations for bowel cancer, maybe even some condition requiring a hysterectomy or other surgery. These interventions, though not pleasant, often seem to bring some kind of closure. Does the body react to the surfacing of memory? – or does the psyche use an illness in the body to assert itself? I don't know.

It was obvious to Dr Gibson that something was

crushing my sciatic nerve and she referred me to an orthopaedic consultant. When I rang the hospital to ask how long it would be before I got an appointment they were sympathetic but not optimistic. 'Let us know if you become incontinent or lose the use of your legs,' they said. When I was finally seen by the consultant he did an immediate scan and reported 'an impressive prolapse at L4'. It was a Friday, and he said he would fit me in at the end of Monday afternoon, giving me a number to ring over the weekend 'if anything happened'.

To my amazement I was not terrified by the prospect of surgery: it was far preferable to the alternatives, and I was desperate to get rid of the pain. Most importantly, Paddy's story of the doctors running towards the target on Frankie's back was now simple nonsense. I no longer believed him – and I dared to trust the doctor.

Not that I was entirely through with Paddy. In early March I had another dream:

> There is a boy of seven or eight (sort of me) who has been persecuted over a long period by some faceless enemies. A second group (with which another 'I' is also loosely associated) want to save him. The first group finally gets him – and the pain is indescribable. The rescuer group still wants to go and get him but cannot face his pain.

My inner persecutor, rescuer and victim were beginning to separate out.

Cocooned in painkillers I was only dimly aware that Pete was also ill at this time: since neither of us was well enough to travel, we commiserated by phone and email. Pete had been sober for seven years. His 'church' – Alcoholics Anonymous – had served him well just as mine had served me well. He was working on a third novel, and was earning more in his job than ever before. Now, however, he had constant headaches, and a series of painful bladder infections which meant he had to drink a lot of water. One day over the phone he described in loving detail the glasses of iced water he would store in the fridge, carefully laced with lemon or mint.

'You sound like an alcoholic talking about a cocktail,' I told him.

'That's right', he answered. 'You've got it.'

After the operation I luxuriated in the coming of spring and nature's affinity with my process of recovery, lying on the couch with the windows open. Jim was at work and I pretended that I was in a nursing home with capable, caring nurses. They would offer me a cup of tea (which I then made myself) or suggest it was time for my walk (which I then took), and praise me for the progress I was making when I returned – all of which did me good. Six weeks later I was signed off by the hospital and phoned Pete to tell him the good news.

'I've just sent you an email', he told me. That afternoon he had walked past St George's and had a massive panic attack outside the parish hall. When he got home he had tried to write down what he could remember about the hall, and sent it to me:

This morning I went round by St George's church hall and I remembered from forty years ago the name of Michael Hamilton in the pantomime singing 'Kicking up leaves.' And his father, Major Hamilton, how forbidding and unfriendly he was in his tweed jacket and moustache, smoking Players with nicotine stained

fingers..... and Mrs Hamilton, his very frail mother ....
I had no memory of these people, but I was moved that
Pete incorporated things I had said:

> *Carolyn remembers Mrs Kowalski going berserk at the*
> *Christmas bazaar and bursting all the children's*
> *balloons.... Who was the woman with the red cheeks?*

He wrote about Jill, our father's Parish Worker. When she
arrived, I had been rather disappointed that she did not
have a bicycle or a chaste blue jacket with a badge on the
lapel, but rode a Lambretta, had a cloud of blonde hair, and
was never far from a powder puff.

> *I remember, wrote Pete, Jill in her rock'n'roll dresses,*
> *stilettos and lovely lipstick, the smell of her face*
> *powder and perfume etc. Her Lambretta. Carolyn*
> *remembers her doing her lipstick and fluffing her hair*
> *in the hall – while the vampires tut-tutted. She was*
> *like a breath of fresh air in the musty coffin of heavy*
> *brogues, tweed skirts and B.O. ...*

> *Carolyn remembered Miss Mullane from our*
> *school teaching us country dancing in the hall, and*
> *how we weren't allowed to get a drink of water from*
> *the tap because her brother had dropped dead from*
> *drinking water after dancing. Providential, I'd say. I*
> *wasn't going to write all this, just a list of names.*

> *Thinking back on those years I get a sensation of*
> *perpetual anxiety and guilt. It was very interesting to*
> *go there with Carolyn in search of the crime scene and*
> *stand in that vicarage garden and look out at the*
> *houses across the road and feel an anxiety close to*
> *terror ...*

> *When puberty flung its baffling and shameful*
> *equations into this mess is it any wonder I found*

release and escape in alcohol. Fucking hell, this is
some heavy fucking therapy.

Was Pete about to begin a memory journey of his own?

There was to be no answer to this question. That evening he had a *grand mal* fit and his life was taken over by headaches, doctor's appointments and a growing exhaustion. Remembering our anxiety about Deidre and driving he went to see his GP to ask if he should still drive after the fit. To his amazement, the GP told him not to worry – 'After all it was only one fit.' He prescribed migraine tablets and referred him for a brain scan, saying it would take several weeks to come through.

Now I was able to drive again I visited Pete and we went out to lunch: the restaurant was near his house but he got lost on the way there. He knew something was very wrong indeed, and when I asked him about the various tests that he was having, he told me, 'They're doing an autopsy to find out why I am still walking around'. There was still no news of when the brain scan would take place.

A few days later Jeanine, his partner, phoned me from her office to say that she could not get any answer from Pete on the home phone. Would I go to their house and see if he was all right? I could not get any answer from him either, and drove straight to London. Pete did answer the door, but it was clearly as much as he could manage, and he sat slumped and silent on the sofa. I sat beside him, perplexed. Was this a physical illness or was it catatonic depression? I asked him how he felt and he managed to say that he was scared he had got a brain tumour. It was our last coherent conversation.

By the time Jeanine came home from work Pete could not even hold a cup of tea without spilling it, and we took him to A and E. When the doctor finally saw him, he was interested in Pete's history of alcoholism and thought he was suffering from depression. Reluctantly, they kept him in, however, and because of the fit they said they would do a brain scan there and then. Within a few days they told us he had an 'aggressive' and inoperable brain tumour, and they expected him to slip into coma and 'fade away quietly' within a few months. That was not Pete's style. He hung on for a year, incontinent, bedridden, mostly in semi-coma, often on the brink of dying – and in receipt of glorious quantities of morphine. Eventually he died in agony, his collapsed veins and clenched teeth preventing the morphine from getting to him.

That is another story, except to say that Pete's long drawn out dying took me to the edge of the abyss and held me there more inexorably than even the return of my story had done. I could not help wondering if his brain had simply closed down on what he could not bear to remember himself. In any case there was no-one left to ask about anything now – only my memories, only my truth.

Richard and Mr O, continued to support me through all this in their own ways. Richard visited Pete more than once in hospital when he was in London for meetings, though there was nothing he could do except sit with him – in just the same way that I had fantasised him sitting with me in the depths of my breakdown.

When Pete died I once again found myself unable to sing the hymns in church. It was Easter time and all the talk of resurrection seemed simply tactless.

Then Mr O. told me he was retiring at the end of the year. I did not feel up to working towards an ending with

228

him and decided to stop seeing him then and there. In a way it felt like an achievement to refuse the ending work and he wrote me a very nice letter accepting my decision. I have often thought since of writing to tell him how much I appreciated our work together, but something has always stopped me. Perhaps that is the secret of my transference to him. What he helped me to achieve was not to have to worry about his feelings before I felt my own feelings – and not to have to express gratitude to someone who had done well the job they were paid for. I needed him simply to have done it because that was what he did.

I was fifty-two, and felt that my life was over – but I did not mind. I knew my story. It had been rich with experience and love in many varieties.

Epilogue
March 2018

ONLY MY TRUTH, from which this book developed, was written in 2011, out of a desire to sum up the story in order to let it go. Seven years later, and nearly two decades since the depression first made itself known, these are my reflections.

It was not a smooth path to recovery. Pete's long, slow dying was followed within six months by the diagnosis of my husband, Jim (a non-smoker), with lung cancer. Kathy and I were able to care for him so he could die at home which to us meant a great deal.

Meanwhile, I had created my own editorial business, which gave me peaceful and interesting work I could do at home. It was not until 2010 – ten years after I first became ill – that I was ready to work with people again. Alongside my editorial business, I built up a new practice as a therapist, supervisor and teacher. My first supervisor, Andrew, was right when he said I had a different job to do for a while: having done that job I brought different things to the work.

Colleagues welcomed me back into the fold, and it was marvellous to find myself still part of the 'family' that has been so much part of my engagement with the outside world in my thirties and forties. Though we were all older – and some, including Andrew and Patricia, had died – the sense of belonging held.

Seven years later I retired, closing my practice gradually and on my own terms, and not on those of a forgotten story and the illness it generated.

Five years after Jim died, I married an old friend who had been widowed for many years. There is little to say about that since happiness is hard to describe. There are grandchildren, and when asked what I would like them to call me, I chose 'Nana'. For decades I had not been able to bring myself to mention her name. Now I have taken it for myself along with all that she gave me.

Sometimes I wonder if my current life is something like what we are supposed to understand by resurrection. It is not so much that I have a second chance or a new life, though that is true, but more that I am living the life I was always trying to live but never quite managed.

During the breakdown I was extraordinarily lucky to have so much support available to me and to be able to afford skilled professional help; there was also the container of my home with Jim and Kathy, and the financial security that went with it, as well as the care and sensitivity of my quixotic brother and many generous friends and colleagues. Also, along with 'Fr Richard', there was the church itself. Though few people there knew what was wrong with me, or even that I was ill, the community and its liturgical cycle provided a secure framework. Without these things I have little doubt I would at some point have needed to be hospitalised.

The experiences I have written about here will always be part of me – but they are only part of my story. I will never have any more evidence about what happened than I do now, but they have found their level in me at last.

REFLECTIONS ON THIS MANUSCRIPT

From this perspective, and after a passage of time, what are my reflections on what is written here?

First, it brings in to sharp relief that the events of my childhood and adolescence happened a very long time ago – and about twenty or thirty years before the seriousness of the sexual abuse of children was properly understood or specific training given in preventing and responding to it. When I was training as a therapist it was a relatively new subject, along with anorexia.

Pete and I were lucky enough to be born into a time of burgeoning consciousness. Though our parents could not protect us, the buck stopped with us, and we were able – in different ways – to work our way through what we had inherited.

In this story there are five people who acted or may have acted as sexual abusers: the verger, my uncle, the hospital doctor, the lodger and Corinna. From this perspective I would say that of these five, only two – the verger and Corinna – radically affected my life. The others are peripheral. This is not to say that what they did was not significant but they added nothing to a pattern that had been passed on in my family probably for generations.

The verger matters because of the violence of his sexual attack and his threats, and the way these broke into what had previously been a trusted environment. The church where he worked was the backdrop to the freedom Pete and I had to wander back and forth between the church and our garden. I enjoyed pottering around with 'Perks', helping with the brass polishing and the Christmas trees, watching him ring the Angelus. All that was shattered in one sudden, unpredictable and violent act.

The deeper significance of what he did, however, lies in my parents' reactions. They were helpless in the face of what had happened and simply did not know how to protect or even reassure me. From that day, also, I was somehow 'spoiled goods' – part of the abusive world in which my mother and father had grown up.

To the twenty-first century mind it may seem astonishing that the verger was not confronted, or fired, or reported to the police or social services – but in the context of my childhood that is not so strange. Freud had exposed and then prevaricated about the sexual abuse of children: at that time society was unable to take in the implications, and by the 1950s not much had changed. People knew these things happen but they believed that small children simply forgot about them: you just got on with life. On the whole people avoided opening the cans of worms that accounted for much of their own depression. In my work I have heard countless stories of lodgers who were not evicted, uncles who were not confronted, priests or teachers allowed to continue in role. Even now, though so many people have been called to account, this goes on.

Corinna

This leaves us with 'Corinna'. My memories of her were never repressed; the problem with Corinna is that she was not a shadowy figure. She was attractive, talented, funny, cultured, a joy to be with. A few months after she died I received a package in the post from Canada. It contained the surplice that she had worn to play the organ in her final post as an organist, and came from a member of the choir. 'I had hoped to wear this myself,' she wrote, 'but I have realised that you are the person who is worthy to have it. Corinna said of you "She is rather good you know," and that must mean you are really something....'

It is at this point that I should confess that the narrative is misleading on the question of what happened to Corinna. It felt too complicated to include my ongoing story with her, so I said that she disappeared from my life after she was fired from my old school. This is not true. She did indeed emigrate, but we kept in close touch, and her letters, which arrived every three weeks for the first year or so, were my lifeblood. She once described my letters to her, which I wrote weekly, as 'galvanising beacons of light in an otherwise phlegmatic world'.

It soon became clear that in her new job she had developed a close bond with an older teacher, Hilda. I do not know if it was ever a sexual relationship, but it was deeply loving and lasted until her death. I am certain that because of that relationship she never abused any more of her pupils. Hilda and I first met about two years after Corinna left England. Corinna's mother had died, and I took her father to visit – the first time he had left the country since the Battle of the Somme. As soon as I met Hilda, I thought, 'So she did want someone like me, after all. I just wasn't old enough.'

In 1987, Corinna wrote to say she had advanced cancer, and I visited her and Hilda for ten days, while Jim and Kathy stayed home. During that visit, Corinna remarked that walking the Pennine Way was the most important thing she had done in her life. Hilda looked a bit surprised. I, of course, treasured the remark. Whatever she meant by that, it was something we had done together. She also said of the cancer (she had refused chemo), 'There is nowhere to go but ahead.' Otherwise, we did not talk much about the past or her impending death. She expressed sadness that there were so many books she would not read now;

she and Hilda had got to the point where when a new book by one of their favourite authors came out, they bought it *and* got it out of the library so they could read and discuss it together.

Back home, I stayed close to both of them by letter and phone calls: it was my first encounter with cancer and what it – and treatment – can do to a person's body. I began to pray, not for Corinna's recovery, but for her and Hilda as they went through this terrible journey. For several painful months, I was constantly aware of them almost like a radio wave inside me. The day Corinna died that sensation came abruptly to an end, an hour or two before Hilda phoned to tell me. It was this experience of spiritual connection that was the beginning of my return to the church.

After Corinna's death, I stayed in touch with Hilda until she too died, in her nineties, some twenty-five years after Corinna. We shared a valuable friendship, and never talked about what had happened between Corinna and me at the beginning.

In spite of marriage and motherhood, years of therapy, the many loving relationships that existed in my life, and the anger I felt about what she had done to me, I was never really free of Corinna. Nor did I want to be.

The #MeToo Campaign

In the autumn of 2017, just as the #MeToo campaign had got underway, my school put out an appeal to old girls inviting them to share experiences of sexual harassment at work for a drama project. I remarked to my husband, 'They might get more than they bargained for,' and indeed they did. A few days later, there in the news was a large picture of the school. Several ex-pupils (all of later generations than me) had got in touch, and subsequently a (male) teacher was asked to leave.

Seeing the picture sent me into shock. It brought right into the present the place which for me belonged in past history, a place which had been hugely important to me, and had quite literally given me an education since I had a full scholarship. It had also, unwittingly, given me Corinna.

I was overwhelmed by a sense of what I had lost through the affair, and got on the phone to say that I, too, had been sexually abused by one of their staff. Within an hour the head mistress called me back. Calmly, I told her what had happened with Corinna – to me and to the others I knew about. Her response was faultless: calm, considerate and kind. Then I told her about *Only My Truth* and said that I wanted to send her the passages relating to the school and Corinna, and receive a response from her. She agreed and her response arrived a few days later. She had clearly taken time to read attentively what I had written, and responded warmly to some particular passages. She also asked permission to share it anonymously with staff and governors who wanted to understand better the effects of sexual abuse. I agreed.

For the first time in fifty years I had taken the story back where it belonged – to the school. It was now theirs to deal with. And for the first time in fifty years I was able to remember and value what I had received from the school: it was not, of course, perfect, but it had changed my life.

Even more importantly, this was the first time I had broken the secret. Over the years I had told the story in many different ways, but always in private: to close friends or family, or in therapy. This was altogether different.

Over the following months, my dreams tracked a

sense of release. And then there was one in which I said very clearly out loud, 'I've played the organ since I was fourteen, but I don't do that anymore.' A fundamental and necessary separation had taken place.

Where does this leave the Corinna story?
What became clear to me through opening up to the school and allowing my story to become part of the institutional problem of sexual abuse, was that Corinna did not know how to manage sex and intimacy. This is not an excuse for the havoc she wreaked in so many young lives, but it does provide some sort of context for understanding her behaviour.

One way to understand the ambivalence this leaves me with is through comments made by other people over the years.

Patricia, my analyst:
During my analysis, which started after Corinna had died, I gave Patricia Corinna's letters to read. She found them terribly sad. 'You loved her so much,' she said, 'but there is no love for you in those letters.' She went on to talk about an older woman who had been very important for her at the same sort of age, but who had cherished her devotion without sexually abusing her. At the time this made me rather cross – she *would* have someone non-abusive, wouldn't she. Nevertheless, it was Patricia, in my mid-thirties, who received all my extreme, transferential, dependent love without retaliation or abuse. She did also love me in a deep, non-sexual way which was new and transformative for me. I learned to love her, too, in this adult non-sexual sense. Years later when I arrived at her

deathbed where her sons were gathered, she said 'All the family are here now.'

Corinna and Hilda:
Could Corinna have done for my adolescent self what Patricia did for my adult self? Her letters occasionally expressed regret: *It is a sad irony that I am the last person who can help you now... I didn't understand that you didn't understand when I said I didn't love you... I had hoped to be someone you could turn to and lean on as you grew up...*

After Corinna died I wrote to Hilda about spending time in retreat and discovering a sense that Corinna had valued my friendship. *Of course she valued your friendship,* Hilda wrote back. And *she always felt angry on your behalf because she felt you had had such a raw deal ....*

Eleanor, a friend:
Eleanor had supported me all through Corinna's dying in the 1980s. When I told her about contacting the school she was horrified. 'But there was so much love!' she exclaimed. The love was all on my side, if you can call something so blind, desperate and needy 'love'. Over the years it did mature, but early on I had no sense of myself separate from Corinna. Nevertheless, after this conversation it took me a while to get over the feeling that by contacting the school I had perhaps betrayed a deep love between Corinna and myself. I also had to ask myself what I would have done if she were still alive; she would now be in her early 80's. I simply do not know the answer to that question.

My closest friend from university:
'It was only when I read your manuscript that I realised how

shocking what Corinna did was. I always thought of her as just Corinna before.'

Another close friend:
'The story as you have written it is important because we don't hear about predatory dykes any more – we lesbians are supposed to be all about love and kindness these days.' I had never thought of Corinna as a predatory dyke, but couldn't deny the description. Yet from her own point of view, she seemed to feel that the girls she seduced were predators on her.

I am not sure what I can conclude from this kaleidoscope of reactions except that while abuse of power is always abuse, and should at all costs be prevented if possible, it can be hard to pin down its motives or indeed its effects.

When I became involved with Corinna I was not ready for sexual relationships – or even close friendships – with people my own age of either sex. She was a bridge to that. Given the state I was in as I reached later adolescence, I cannot help thinking that if it had not been her it would have been someone else. I was a sitting duck. And at that age I am not sure I would have coped with someone responding to my needy love while maintaining proper boundaries.

This is not to say there is nothing to forgive, but my anger is much less than it was. I learned a great deal from her musically and in other ways, and still value the new horizons she opened up for me. I regret that for so many years these things were shrouded in pain, but I have been able to appropriate them in the end.

I am one of the lucky ones: no longer an easy target

for abuse. Long after their deaths, I am at peace with my parents. I do not even feel like a survivor any more. I am aware of my history, but it is overlaid with the richness of my current life. I am simply myself.

A RECENT ENCOUNTER

A few months ago, waiting for a concert to begin, I started chatting with a young woman sitting next to me. She was somehow familiar. It was not that I had met her before but her manner and style of speaking reminded me of a certain type of churchgoer – young, committed, enthusiastic. It turned out that she was visiting her family for a few days; she lived not far from where I grew up and was indeed a churchgoer, though not at St George's where my father had been the vicar.

I asked her if she knew St George's and she did. She had a friend who went there. What a marvellous building it was, she said. I found myself saying, 'My father was vicar of that church when I was a child. I grew up in that vicarage behind the church.'

'Oh', she said, 'that enormous house with the huge garden alongside the church grounds.'

'Yes – that's it.'

'What an idyllic childhood.'

I smiled and nodded. And then the concert began.